Principles of Pharmacoeconomics

J. Lyle Bootman, Ph.D.
Raymond J. Townsend, Pharm.D.
William F. McGhan, Pharm.D., Ph.D.

W HARVEY WHITNEY BOOKS COMPANY

HARVEY WHITNEY BOOKS COMPANY
4906 Cooper Rd., P.O. Box 42696, Cincinnati, OH 45242 USA

Library of Congress Catalog Card Number: 90-070693
International Standard Book Number: 0-929375-02-5

Table of Contents

Preface

During the next decade, the development of new drugs will be stimulated by an increased understanding of disease processes and the application of biotechnology discoveries. The use of these new clinical agents in practice will be increasingly determined by not only their effectiveness, but also the cost of the technology. In essence, the rising costs of healthcare will force decisions to be made regarding both the effectiveness of the technology and the overall cost implications. Therefore, the purpose of this book is to present various techniques, tools, and strategies to evaluate the economic contribution of specific drug therapies at a policy level and for individual patient needs. This information is relevant for researchers, practitioners, and students of the science.

Additionally, it is our hope that this book will further stimulate pharmacists, physicians, and others to generate more pharmacoeconomic research in order to adequately apply the results to the prevention and treatment of disease.

This book could not have been put together without the administrative assistance of the University of Arizona College of Pharmacy staff, especially Sandra Rogers and Debra Ciszek-Olson. As is customary for all of his word processing needs, Dr. Bootman is deeply indebted to one of the most dedicated staff at the University of Arizona, Daina Wasson. Finally, we would like to thank our families, colleagues, and friends for their support, love, and especially their understanding as we completed this task.

J. Lyle Bootman
Raymond J. Townsend
William F. McGhan

Contributing Authors

Judith T. Barr, Sc.D.
Associate Professor and Director
Master of Health Professions Program
College of Pharmacy and
   Allied Health Professions
Northeastern University
Boston, Massachusetts
Chapter 7

J. Lyle Bootman, Ph.D.
Professor and Acting Dean
Executive Director
Center for Pharmaceutical Economics
College of Pharmacy
University of Arizona
Tucson, Arizona
Chapters 1 and 9

Elizabeth A. Chrischilles, Ph.D.
Assistant Professor
Department of Preventive Medicine and
   Environmental Health
College of Medicine
University of Iowa
Iowa City, Iowa
Chapter 5

JoLaine R. Draugalis, Ph.D.
Assistant Professor
Center for Pharmaceutical Economics
College of Pharmacy
University of Arizona
Tucson, Arizona
Chapter 8

Jean Paul Gagnon, Ph.D.
Director, Industry Affairs
Marion Merrell Dow Inc.
Kansas City, Missouri
Chapter 2

Ronald W. Hansen, Ph.D.
Associate Dean for Academic Affairs
The William E. Simon Graduate School of
   Business Administration
University of Rochester
Rochester, New York
Chapter 4

Deborah S. Kitz, Ph.D.
Executive Director
Abington Surgical Center
Willow Grove, Pennsylvania
Chapter 6

Lon N. Larson, Ph.D.
Associate Professor
Center for Pharmaceutical Economics
College of Pharmacy
University of Arizona
Tucson, Arizona
Chapter 3

William F. McGhan, Pharm.D., Ph.D.
Professor and Executive Director
Institute for Pharmaceutical Economics
Chairman
Department of Pharmacy Practice and
   Pharmacy Administration
Philadelphia College of Pharmacy and
   Science
Philadelphia, Pennsylvania
Chapter 1

Jane T. Osterhaus, Ph.D.
Assistant Director, Clinical
   Applications
Glaxo Inc.
Research Triangle Park, North Carolina
Chapter 8

Gerald E. Schumacher, Pharm.D., Ph.D.
Professor
College of Pharmacy and
   Allied Health Professions
Northeastern University
Boston, Massachusetts
Chapter 7

Raymond J. Townsend, Pharm.D.
Director, Medical Marketing
Glaxo Inc.
Research Triangle Park, North Carolina
Chapter 1

1

1

Introduction to Pharmacoeconomics

J. Lyle Bootman
Raymond J. Townsend
William F. McGhan

I n 1988, the U.S. spent $560 billion on healthcare, representing slightly over 11.1 percent of the nation's gross national product.[1] In addition, the Health Care Financing Administration projected that the nation's health expenditures would reach $647.3 billion in 1990.[1] Drugs and pharmacy dispensing charges accounted for $34 billion, or less than eight percent of the 1987 total healthcare expenditures.[2] U. S. consumers pay directly personally for much of their medication cost. Private health insurance and government programs cover a growing portion of drug expenditures, but approximately 58 percent of drug costs are still paid directly by consumers.[1] The cost of pharmaceuticals and pharmacy services have, therefore, become an important issue to patients, third-party payers, and governments. Today, and in the future, it is necessary to scientifically value the costs and consequences of drug therapy.

The basic value of drug therapy to prescribers and patients in the U.S. is evidenced by the increased therapeutic use of prescriptions. In 1988, community pharmacists dispensed approximately 1.7 billion prescriptions.[3] From the 1950s to 1980, the number of prescriptions dispensed per person per year in the U.S. has increased from 2.4 to 6.8. The nation's hospitals provide approximately $5 billion worth of drugs and drug products to hospitalized patients.[4] Drugs available without prescription also serve an important role in the healthcare of the U.S. population. Use of nonprescription drugs in this country has greatly increased. Since the 1950s, the sales of OTC drugs have increased from $700 million to approximately $8.1 billion in 1989.[4,5] These figures may be indicative of the value and perceived benefit that society attributes to medications. Most economists would acknowledge that a crude, lower-bound estimate of the value and benefits of drugs to consumers is the amount they spend on these products.

3

Pharmaceuticals and other therapeutic interventions have contributed to the important progress being made in the health status of the U.S. population. Life expectancy, which continues to increase, is currently at 78.3 years for women and 71.5 years for men. Corresponding to the introduction of new drug entities during the past two decades, the mortality rates for several diseases have declined substantially. Heart disease mortality declined by 7.5 percent from 1982 to 1987.[1]

Drugs account for only about five percent of the expenditures in hospital budgets, but drug therapy plays a crucial role in the efficient treatment of hospitalized patients. An average hospitalized patient receives six to eight different drugs on a typical day. Effective drug therapy helps to explain partially why the mean length of stay in hospitals has decreased to 6.8 days in 1988.[6]

Despite the general evidence supporting the use of pharmaceuticals, very little information actually exists that compiles and analyzes the actual costs and benefits attributed to specific drug therapies. A primary reason is the lack of defined economic methodologies available to evaluate medical interventions. Perhaps the current focus on reducing expenditures of pharmaceuticals and pharmacy services to save costs to the total healthcare system is inappropriate. A purpose of this book is to present economic methodologies that may be employed not only to evaluate drug therapy, but also put them in perspective with other related healthcare expenditures.

Definition of Pharmacoeconomics Research

Pharmacoeconomics has been defined as "the description and analysis of the costs of drug therapy to healthcare systems and society."[7] Pharmacoeconomic research identifies, measures, and compares the costs (i.e., resources consumed) and consequences of pharmaceutical products and services. The research methods related to cost-minimization, cost-effectiveness, cost-benefit, cost-of-illness, cost-utility, decision-analysis, and quality-of-life (QOL) assessments are included within this framework. In essence, pharmacoeconomic analysis employs tools for examining the impact (desirable and undesirable) of alternative drug therapies and other medical interventions. Some of these terms are defined below:

Cost-benefit analysis: costs and consequences are simultaneously measured in terms of dollars.

Cost-effectiveness analysis: costs and consequences are simultaneously measured; effectiveness in terms of obtaining a specified objective and cost in monetary terms.

Cost-utility analysis: consequences are measured in terms of quality of life, willingness to pay, or preference of one intervention to another.

Cost-minimization analysis: costs are analyzed and compared where two or more interventions have been demonstrated or assumed to be equivalent in terms of the outcome or consequence.

Cost-of-illness evaluation: identifies and evaluates the direct and indirect costs of a particular disease.

Questions that pharmacoeconomics may help to address are as follows: What drugs should be included on the hospital formulary? What is the best drug for a particular patient? What is the best drug for a pharmaceutical manufacturer to develop? Which drug delivery system is the best for this hospital? How do these two clinical pharmacy services compare? Which drugs should be included in the Medicaid formulary? What is the cost per quality year of life extended by this drug? Will patient QOL be improved by a particular drug-therapy decision? What is the best drug for this particular disease? What are the patient outcomes of various treatment modalities?

In essence, pharmacoeconomic analysis employs important tools for examining the impact of drug therapy and related medical interventions.

Overview of Pharmacoeconomic Methodologies

The purpose of this section is to acquaint the reader with the basic methodological approaches regarding the economic evaluation of drug therapy. By definition, pharmacoeconomic evaluations include any study designed to assess the costs (i.e., resources consumed) and consequences of alternative therapies. This includes such methodologies labeled as cost-benefit, cost-utility, and cost-effectiveness. Each of these methodologies is discussed in more depth in later chapters. Both review articles and studies that have actually applied these techniques to healthcare evaluations may assist the interested reader in becoming more aware of the role of these tools.[8-31] The evaluation mechanisms delineated were often helpful in demonstrating the cost-impact of innovative treatments, therefore granting them greater acceptance by healthcare providers, administrators, and the public.

COST-BENEFIT ANALYSIS

Cost-benefit analysis (CBA) is not a new concept used in evaluating health interventions. Basically, CBA is a tool that can be used to improve the decision-making process in allocation of funds to healthcare and other programs.[32-34] The general concept of CBA is not overly complicated; however, many technical considerations require a certain degree of explanation and interpretation in order to understand how CBA can be or has been applied.

CBA evolved from the need to ascertain estimates of the costs and resultant benefits of public investment projects. Expenditures for healthcare should produce net social benefits for the public. CBA techniques can be applied to make such resource allocation decisions in the healthcare field. Several economists state that medical care is both an investment good and a consumption good.[35,36] When considered as an investment good, medical care is an investment in human capital. In economic terms, the value of a person's lifetime productivity or earnings is the appropriate measure of the potential benefit from investment in human capital. As Pigou points out, "The most important investment of all is the investment in health, intelligence, and character of the people."[37]

A major function in any planning process is the formulation of alternative ways to achieve desired objectives and of criteria to choose among the alternatives. Many times, decisions are made on the basis of intuition and personal judgment. CBA, by requiring precise definitions and objectives, identification of criteria for judging results, and quantification of the results of each alternative through formal exposition of alternatives and examination of the effects of assumptions and uncertainties, provides a more solid basis for decision making. Prest and Turvey stated that "an important advantage of cost-benefit study is that it forces those responsible to quantify costs and benefits, as far as possible, rather than rest content with vague, qualitative judgments or personal hunches."[38]

CBA consists of identifying all the benefits that accrue from the program or intervention and converting them into dollars in the year in which they will occur. This stream of benefit dollars is then discounted to its equivalent present value at the selected interest rate. On the other side of the equation, all program costs are identified and allocated through a specific year and, again, the costs are discounted to their present value at the same interest rate. If all relevant factors remain constant, the program with the largest present value of benefits minus costs is the best in terms of its economic value.

Ideally, all benefits and costs resulting from the program should be included. This presents considerable difficulty, especially on the benefits side of the equation, since many benefits are either difficult to measure, difficult to convert to dollars, or both. For example, benefits such as improved patient comfort, improved patient satisfaction with the healthcare system, improved working conditions for the physician, and so on, are not only difficult to measure, but are extremely difficult to convert into dollars. This problem has been addressed by many researchers in health economics and has not been completely resolved. Much of the work in CBA has attempted to solve this problem, but an acceptable solution has yet to be found. Generally, the analyst or researcher will convert as many benefits as possible into monetary units. The remaining variables are labeled as "intangible benefits" and left to decision makers to include in their final deliberations.

COST-EFFECTIVENESS ANALYSIS

Edward S. Quade of the Rand Corporation defines cost-effectiveness as a technique "designed to assist a decision maker in identifying a preferred choice among possible alternatives."[39] Generally, cost-effectiveness is defined as a "series of analytical and mathematical procedures which aid in the selection of a course of action from various alternative approaches."[40-42]

As stated by Shepard and Thompson, cost-effectiveness analysis (CEA) is a way of summarizing the health benefits and resources used by competing healthcare programs so that policy makers can choose among them. Essentially, program/treatment costs are summarized in one total figure and program effects (benefits) into a second total figure. Decisions then are based on the effectiveness to cost ratios between the competing programs. An alternative definition is that CEA is a method to determine which program/treatment accomplishes a given objective at minimum cost.[43]

Requirements included in CEA studies are that: (1) the optimal alternative (not necessarily the least costly) for accomplishing an objective is possible, (2) at least two alternatives are possible, and (3) cost-effectiveness need not be cost reduction, but rather an optimizing process.

Cost-effectiveness methodology requires that clear, articulate objectives be set. Following this process, it is recommended that five types of measurement be made for each alternative: (1) outcome/impact, (2) operation use, (3) personnel and equipment needed, (4) cost factors and discount rates, and (5) costs.

Generally, CEA has been applied to health matters where the program's inputs can be readily measured in dollars, but the program's outputs are more appropriately stated in terms of the health improvement created (e.g., life-years extended). Weinstein and Stason provided an excellent explanation of the use of CEA for practicing physicians and physician administrators. This article is highly recommended for those interested in a more detailed discussion.[10]

An important point to be considered in both CBA and CEA is that a program/treatment providing a high benefit (effectiveness) to cost ratio in terms of value to society as a whole may not be valued in the same way by other members of society. For example, drug therapy that reduced the number of patient-days in an acute-care institution may be positive from a third-party payer's point of view, but not necessarily from the view of the institution's administrator who operated under a fixed level of revenue and who depended upon a fixed number of patient-days to meet expenses. What is viewed as cost-beneficial for society as a whole may be viewed differently by plan sponsors, administrators, healthcare providers, governmental agencies, or patients. One must consider whose interests are to be taken into account when using CBA and CEA.

COST-MINIMIZATION

When two or more interventions are examined and demonstrated or assumed to be equivalent in terms of a given outcome or consequence, costs associated with each intervention may be examined and compared. This typical cost-analysis is referred to as cost-minimization analysis. An example of this type of analysis with regard to drug therapy may be the evaluation of two generically equivalent drugs in which the outcome has been proven to be equal; however, the acquisition and administration costs of the two drugs may be significantly different.

COST-UTILITY

In examining Table 1, one can better appreciate the subtle differences between the techniques discussed to this point. Cost-utility analysis is an economic tool in which the intervention consequence is measured in terms of patient preference or quality of the healthcare outcome. It is much the same as cost-effectiveness analysis with the added dimension of a particular point of view—most often that of the patient. Quite often the results of a cost-utility analysis are expressed in intervention cost per quality-adjusted-life-year (QALY) gained, or changes in QOL measurement for a given intervention cost.

COST-OF-ILLNESS EVALUATIONS

Examination of the overall (direct and indirect) costs of a particular disease to a defined population is referred to as a cost-of-illness evaluation. This economic methodology attempts to define, in a macroeconomic sense, all of the costs associated with a particular disease. Several studies have attempted to examine the cost of various disease states. Macroeconomic presentations on the economic costs of specific illnesses have been published, expanding on the costs of illness and death in the U.S. using the cost-of-illness.[36,41] Table 2 illustrates the total cost-of-illness for selected diseases.[44]

It is important to understand the difference between direct and indirect costs of illness. Direct costs represent expenditures for prevention, detection, treatment, rehabilitation, research, training, and capital investment in medical facilities. Indirect costs are related to morbidity costs from lost work days and mortality costs, which refers to the income foregone by an individual due to death.

Table 1. Pharmacoeconomic Methodologies

Methodology	Cost Measurement Unit	Outcome Unit
Cost-benefit	dollars	dollars
Cost-effectiveness	dollars	natural units (life-years gained, mg/dL blood sugar, mm Hg blood pressure)
Cost-minimization	dollars	assume to be equivalent in comparative groups
Cost-utility	dollars	quality-adjusted life-year or other utilities

Table 2. Total Costs (Direct and Indirect) of Selected Illnesses[43]

Illness	Cost ($ billions)
Circulatory system diseases	80
Digestive system diseases	56
Neoplasms	40
Respiratory diseases	30
Mental disorders	25

If one successfully identifies both the direct and indirect costs of a particular disease, then conducting an economic evaluation of a particular preventive intervention enables one to calculate the benefit-to-cost ratio. For example, let's assume we conducted a study to estimate the total cost-of-illness (direct plus indirect) of osteoporosis to be $5 billion. Additionally, a prevention program was implemented across the U.S. that was estimated to cost $1.8 billion. The overall savings to the U.S. would be $3.2 billion, which may be determined by estimating the total cost of the disease minus the cost of the intervention. Such an approach has been used for evaluating many infectious diseases such as tuberculosis, poliomyelitis, and smallpox.

Pharmacoeconomics and Drug Development

In 1988 the pharmaceutical industry spent over $6.5 billion for the development of new drugs; in 1989, it is estimated to be $7.3 billion.[45] This figure represents approximately 16 percent of sales. This certainly is higher compared with other industries. It has been estimated that it takes $125 million and ten years to bring a new drug to the market. The process by which a drug is evaluated and developed for the marketplace is illustrated in Figure 1.

A major question arises as to when is the ideal time to conduct pharmaceutical studies. Figure 1 illustrates the development stages of a new drug. Pharmacoeconomic studies may be planned and conducted at the clinical development stage and at the Phase IV stage of postmarketing. Another thought is that basic research and development activities may be partially guided by preliminary pharmacoeconomic analyses. Therefore, studies may need to be conducted at several stages of pharmaceutical research. The following is a summary of the research activity for each phase.

PHASE I TRIALS

The objective of the initial clinical trials (Phase I) is to determine the toxicity profile of the drug in humans. The first Phase I trials usually consist of administration of single, conservative doses to a small number of healthy volunteers. The effects of increasing the size and number of daily doses are evaluated until toxic effects occur or the likely therapeutic dosage is substantially exceeded. It is during this stage that cost-of-illness studies should be accomplished to aid in the decision to further develop the drug and to gather background data for future pharmacoeconomic evaluations.

PHASE II TRIALS

In Phase II trials, the drug is administered to a limited number of patients with the target disease. Patients without complicating, coexisting medical conditions are preferred for these trials. This reduces the number of variables that could confound analysis of the drug's activity and permits the potential therapeutic benefit of the new drug to be more clearly demonstrated.

Even in carefully selected patients, however, demonstrating the efficacy of a new drug is neither easy nor certain. To provide unequivocal evidence of the drug's therapeutic benefit, it is necessary to compare its effectiveness with that of standard medically accepted treatments or, where ethically appropriate, with a placebo. These comparisons also are used to establish the optimal dosage range for therapeutic activity of the new drug. During this phase, cost-of-disease studies can begin or continue, as well as preliminary development of QOL instruments.

PHASE III TRIALS

In Phase III trials, larger numbers of patients are given the new drug in the established dosage range and the final dosage form. This larger sample size refines the knowledge gained during Phase II and helps identify patients who might have rare reactions to the drug. Patient selection is still closely supervised and some patients with coexisting medical problems are intentionally included to assess complications in the drug's use. If appropriate, patients with varying severities of the target disease are included to determine the new drug's scope of action.

The drug's pharmacokinetic profile—how much of it gets into the body and how quickly, how it is metabolized and eliminated, the effects of multiple doses on drug concentrations, and the relationship between drug concentration and therapeutic activity—is extensively evaluated in patients and healthy volunteers.

Discussion, planning, and implementation of pharmacoeconomic studies during this level of research are important. The prospective clinical study that has incorporated a pharmacoeconomic study is close to the ideal situation. Critics of these studies claim that pharmacoeconomic evaluations will hinder the new drug application process. Advocates of pharmacoeconomic evaluation correctly note that, unless a new drug treatment has no alternatives and is truly a breakthrough, the value of using it must be scientifically studied.

PHASE IV

During the postmarketing phase (Phase IV), prospective and retrospective pharmacoeconomic studies can be designed and conducted to support the use of the drug. Postmarketing pharmacoeconomic studies are extremely important in that they allow one to study the costs and consequences of drug therapy without altered interventions that occur in strictly controlled clinical trials.

Relationships Between Economic Evaluations and Clinical Trials

As previously indicated, clinical trials are used to evaluate the efficacy and safety of therapies. The relationship between economic evaluations and clinical

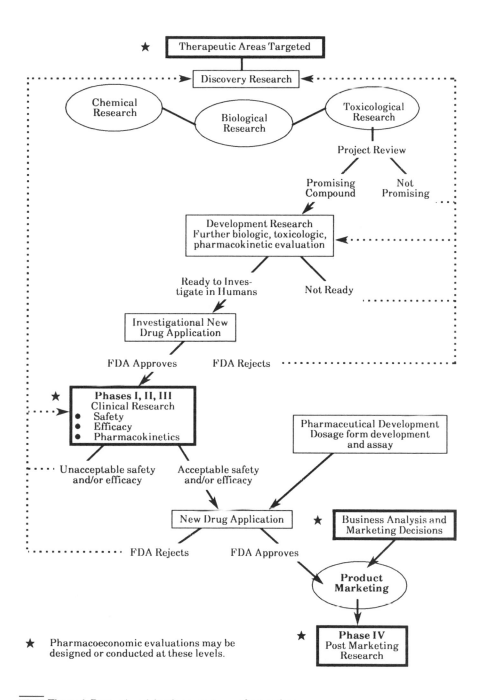

Figure 1. Research and development stages of a new drug.

trials are threefold: (1) the pharmacoeconomic evaluation may be a secondary objective of a trial designed primarily for safety and efficacy, (2) the pharmacoeconomic evaluation may be the principal purpose of a clinical trial, or (3) a pharmacoeconomic evaluation may be done retrospectively on clinical data obtained in previous trials.

A pharmacoeconomic evaluation has a different focus than the traditional clinical trial in two respects. First, the economic evaluation is more concerned about extrapolating to what happens in "real life" than under controlled conditions. In other words, the economic study is more interested in effectiveness (what happens under actual conditions of use) rather than efficacy (what occurs in ideal conditions).

Second, the economic study attempts to measure different outcomes. While the clinical trial focuses on medical indicators (e.g., blood pressure), the economic study is designed to measure the effects on resource consumption, productivity, and/or QOL.

As a consequence of these differences, the intensive clinical monitoring that is part of a clinical trial is not necessarily desirable in the economic trial. However, other design aspects of a clinical trial are often critically important in the economic evaluation (e.g., specific patient selection criteria, random assignment, "blinded" clinicians and patients).

Because pharmacoeconomic data are becoming increasingly important to practitioners making drug formulary decisions, it is important to have these data as swiftly as possible after the drug receives FDA approval. To do this, discussion and planning for pharmacoeconomic evaluation should begin during the early stages of the drug's development. Studies designed to evaluate the costs of disease and current treatments can begin early in Stages I and II. QOL instrument development and validation can also be conducted simultaneously with the clinical trials. Cost-effectiveness and costs associated with toxicities and treatment failures can initially begin in Phases II or III; however, because Phase II trials are rigidly controlled, often much of the pharmacoeconomic data profile of a drug is generated after the drug is marketed. Once a drug is marketed (Phase IV), either prospective or retrospective pharmacoeconomic studies may be designed and conducted utilizing pharmacoepidemiological and pharmacoeconomic methodologies.

Pharmacoepidemiology studies are employed frequently to further study the efficacy and safety of drugs at the Phase IV level of drug research. Epidemiological data with regard to the disease and treatment under investigation can yield highly important information in the economic evaluation of a specific drug therapy. Understanding the natural progression of the disease and treatment enables one to estimate variables that may have pharmacoeconomic implications with regard to the cost of illness and QOL.

In short, an economic evaluation may be added as a component to a clinical trial with the goal to monitor or estimate:

1. Resource consumption: health services and other (direct costs and benefits)
2. Lost productivity through morbidity and/or premature death (indirect costs and benefits)
3. QOL or willingness to pay

General Steps in Designing an Economic Evaluation

There are several steps in designing the pharmacoeconomic study that should be addressed for the specific economic methodology (e.g., cost-effectiveness versus cost-benefit). To illustrate this, the steps associated with CEA are listed below.

Step 1: Prior to incorporating pharmacoeconomic evaluation into any clinical trial, the investigator must first establish the perspective from which to evaluate the various costs and benefits. That is, will the costs and consequences be those of society, specific patients, a third-party payer, health-maintenance organizations, or hospitals? Depending on the perspective an investigator takes, the methodology may vary greatly.

Step 2: Describe/specify the clinical treatment alternatives. The alternatives included in a pharmacoeconomic evaluation should be those actually available to the decision-maker.

Step 3: For each treatment alternative, specify the possible outcomes (i.e., patient pathways) and their probabilities. This can be retrospective, using information from clinical studies, medical literature, and/or expert panels. It also can be a product of a current clinical trial. The pathways often can be presented clearly in the form of decision trees or similar diagrams.

Step 4: Specify and monitor the healthcare resources consumed in each pathway. The resources include: drugs, physician services, hospital "hotel" and ancillary services, laboratory tests, and so on. This can be done retrospectively or concurrently with a clinical trial. If this is done retrospectively, each patient pathway is described in terms of the healthcare resources that are likely to be consumed. If concurrent with a clinical trial, the artificial use of services (i.e., those required by the trial's protocol) must be considered.

The perspective of the study (e.g., insurer, hospital, society) affects the resources that are included. For instance, a diagnosis-related-group-paid hospital is not concerned with the increased intensity of nursing home care that may be associated with shorter hospital stays.

Step 5: Assign dollar values to each resource consumed. In drug studies, hospital services require special attention because of their relative magnitude. Also, drug prices need to be selected carefully because of their availability.

Step 6: Specify and monitor non-healthcare resources consumed in each pathway. Generally, this is not a concern in drug studies. These resources, such as the economic impact a patient's treatment has on the family, often are difficult to measure. They should be estimated or at least noted and brought into discussion as a caveat when reporting the results of the study.

Step 7: Specify the unit of effectiveness. The appropriate unit depends on the disease/condition and the results of treatment. Some possibilities are: patient lives saved, years of life added, or reduction in morbidity attributed to the disease. (These data are derived from the clinical portion of the trial.)

Step 8: Specify other noneconomic attributes of the alternatives (e.g., pain, adverse effects). These may be difficult to quantify and may lead to employing QOL determination and cost-utility analysis.

Step 9: Analyze the data employing the appropriate pharmacoeconomic methodology (e.g., CEA, cost-minimization analysis). The appropriate analysis will be determined by how the study was set up, the perspective, and the type and quality of the data gathered.

Step 10: Conduct a sensitivity analysis. Ratios are recalculated, using different values for uncertain items. Sensitivity analysis essentially defines a range of confidence for the results of the study.

Challenges for Pharmacoeconomic Research

In the future we will be routinely challenged to do pharmacoeconomic research; however, just doing it will not solve all of the problems all of the time. To be useful, appropriate pharmacoeconomic evaluations must be tailored to the specific problem and decision at hand. Our challenge, therefore, begins with looking beyond the obvious and easy solutions. Cost-minimization analysis is useful when comparing interventions with identical outcomes, but this can be the exception rather than the rule for many clinical applications outside of true generic substitution. CBA would, at first glance, be the answer to more complex problems, in that it would allow for evaluation of various interventions with multiple and dissimilar outcomes. Here, too, one must be careful to note the pitfalls and challenges associated with converting all of the benefits to monetary terms (how does one go about placing a monetary value on reduced blood pressure or insulin control?). Allowing consequences to remain in natural and measurable terms means that CEA may be appropriate for many problems and help with many decisions when the outcomes of the interventions are measured in the same terms. But what about the patient and how the various treatments affect daily living and QOL? Should decisions be made strictly on getting the most clinical outcome for the dollar spent? Perhaps then, it is cost-utility analysis, taking into account patient preference and QOL, that should be the gold standard of pharmacoeconomic research; alas, here too, there are problems of measuring QOL and preference in a changing world.

Present and future controversies surrounding pharmacoeconomic research also include arguments for methodologies of valuations and discounting. What is the most appropriate perspective to take when valuing costs and consequences: the patient, the physician, or perhaps the third-party payer? What about ethics— will we be able to justify our decisions solely on the numbers obtained through scientific research?

The challenges of pharmacoeconomic research are inexhaustible; many of them are addressed in this book. The real challenge, however, is not in identifying the tools of pharmacoeconomic research, but rather in discovering how and when to use them.

Summary

The overall costs of medical and pharmaceutical care continue to rise. The added value to society, individual healthcare institutions, and patients as weighed against the costs has not been well established. The problem has become increasingly difficult to address because of the lack of understanding of methodologies to evaluate new and existing drug therapy. The remaining chapters of this text provide in-depth information on specific methodologies employed in pharmacoeconomic investigations.

References

1. Sourcebook of health insurance data. Washington, DC: Health Insurance Association of America, 1989:39.

2. PMA newsletter 1989;*31*(28): July 24.

3. Annual Rx survey. *Am Druggist* 1989;*199*(5):36-42.

4. Manasse HR. Medication use in an imperfect world: drug misadventuring as an issue of public policy. *Am J Hosp Pharm* 1988;*46*:929-44.

5. Your place in the race for OTC/HBA sales. *Drug Topics* 1990;*134*(8):30-44.

6. Digest for hospital pharmacy. Indianapolis: Eli Lilly, 1989:4.

7. Townsend RJ. Post-marketing drug research and development. *Drug Intell Clin Pharm* 1987;*21*:134-6.

8. McGhan W, Rowland C, Bootman JL. Cost-benefit and cost-effectiveness: methodologies for evaluating innovative pharmaceutical services. *Am J Hosp Pharm* 1978;*35*:133-40.

9. Bootman JL, Rowland C, Wertheimer A. Cost-benefit analysis: a research tool for evaluating innovative health programs. *Eval Health Prof* 1979;*2*:129-54.

10. Weinstein MC, Stason WB. Foundations of cost/effectiveness analysis for health and medical practices. *N Engl J Med* 1977;*296*:716-21.

11. Acton J. Measuring the monetary value of life-saving programs. *Law Contemp Probl* 1976; *40*:46-72.

12. Bootman JL, Wertheimer A, Zaske D, Rowland C. Individualizing gentamicin dosage regimens on burn patients with gram-negative septicemia: a cost-benefits analysis. *J Pharm Sci* 1979;*68*:267-72.

13. Bootman JL, Zaske D, Wertheimer AL, Rowland C. Individualization of aminoglycoside dosage regimens: a cost analysis. *Am J Hosp Pharm* 1979;*36*:368-70.

14. Strange PV, Sumner AT. Predicting treatment costs and life expectancy for end-stage renal disease. *N Engl J Med* 1978;*298*:372-8.
15. Cretin S. Cost/benefit analysis of treatment and prevention of myocardial infarction. *Health Serv Res* 1977;*12*:174-89.
16. Mattsson W, Glynning I, Carlsson B, Mauritzon SE. Cancer chemotherapy in advanced malignant disease: a cost-benefit analysis. *Acta Radiol Oncol* 1979;*18*:509-20.
17. Goldschmidt PG. A cost/effectiveness model for evaluating health care programs: application to drug abuse treatment. *Inquiry* 1976;*13*:29-47.
18. Estershan RJ Jr, Vogal VG, Fortner CL, Shapiro HM, Wiernik PH. Cost analysis of leukemia treatment: a problem-oriented approach. *Cancer* 1976;*37*:646-52.
19. Stason WB, Weinstein MC. Allocation of resources to manage hypertension. *N Engl J Med* 1977;*297*:732-9.
20. Adams JG. The societal impact of pharmaceuticals: an overview. Washington, DC: Pharmaceutical Manufacturers Association, 1983.
21. Weisbrod BA, Huston JH. Benefits and costs of human vaccines in developed countries: an evaluative survey. Washington, DC: Pharmaceutical Manufacturers Association, 1983.
22. Haaga JG. Cost-effectiveness and cost-benefit analysis of immunization programs in developing countries: a review of the literature. Washington, DC: Pharmaceutical Manufacturers Association, 1983.
23. Wagner JL. Economic evaluations of medicines: a review of the literature. Washington, DC: Pharmaceutical Manufacturers Association, 1983.
24. Dao TD. Cost-benefit and cost-effectiveness analysis of pharmaceutical intervention. Washington, DC: Pharmaceutical Manufacturers Association, 1983.
25. Vinokur A. The role of survey research in the assessment of health and quality-of-life outcomes of pharmaceutical interventions. Washington, DC: Pharmaceutical Manufacturers Association, 1983.
26. Little AD. Beta-blocker reduction of mortality and reinfarction rate in survivors of myocardial infarctions: a cost-benefit study. Washington, DC: Pharmaceutical Manufacturers Association, 1983.
27. Little AD. Use of a beta blocker in the treatment of glaucoma: a cost-benefit study. Washington, DC: Pharmaceutical Manufacturers Association, 1983.
28. Little AD. Use of beta blockers in the treatment of angina: a cost-benefit study. Washington, DC: Pharmaceutical Manufacturers Association, 1983.
29. Dao TD. Cost-benefit and cost-effectiveness analysis of drug therapy. *Am J Hosp Pharm* 1985;*42*:791-802.
30. Drummond MF, Stoddart GL, Torrance GW. Methods for the economic evaluation of health care programmes. New York: Oxford University Press, 1986.
31. Guyatt G, Drummond M, Feeny D, et al. Guidelines for the clinical and economic evaluation of health care technologies. *Soc Sci Med* 1986;*22*:393-408.
32. Bryers F, Hawthorne VM. Screening for mild hypertension: costs and benefits. *J Epidemiol Commun Health* 1978;*32*:171-4.
33. Klarman H. Application of cost/benefit analysis to health services and the special case of technological innovation. *Int J Health Serv Res* 1974;*4*:325-52.
34. Klarman H. Present status of cost-benefit analysis in the health field. *Am J Public Health* 1967;*57*:1948-58.
35. Smith W. Cost/effectiveness and cost/benefit for public health programs. *Public Health Rep* 1968;*83*:899-906.

36. Mushkin S, d'Accolings F. Economic cost of disease and injury. *Public Health Rep* 1959; *74*:338-45.

37. Pigou AC. Socialism versus capitalism. London: Macmillan, 1947:129.

38. Prest AR, Turvey R. Cost-benefits analysis: a survey. *Econ J* 1965; *75*:683-735.

39. Quade ES. Introduction and overview. In: Goldman TA, ed. Cost-effectiveness analysis. New York: Praeger, 1967:1.

40. Vracin RA. Decision models for capital investment and financing decisions in hospitals. *Health Serv Res* 1980;*15*:35-52.

41. Rice DP. Measurement and application of illness costs. *Public Health Rep* 1969;*84*:95-101.

42. Crystal R, Brewster A. Cost-benefit and cost-effectiveness analysis in the health field: an introduction. *Inquiry* 1966;*3*:3-13.

43. Shepard DS, Thompson MS. First principles of cost-effectiveness analysis in health. *Public Health Rep* 1979;*94*:535-44.

44. Donabedian A, Axelrod SJ, Wyszewianski L, Lichtenstein RL. Medical care chartbook, 8th ed. Ann Arbor, MI: Health Administration Press, 1986:114.

45. A year of innovation: the pharmaceutical industry in 1989. Pharmaceutical Manufacturers Association, 1989:15.

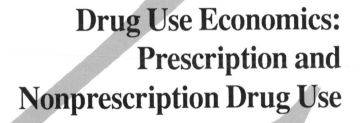

2

Drug Use Economics: Prescription and Nonprescription Drug Use

Jean Paul Gagnon

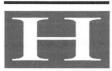ealthcare providers in the 1980s have witnessed a surge in new prescription product introductions similar to the one that occurred in the 1950s. The number of new products released in 1989 was in the double digits, as it has been since 1982. Moreover, more than 15 percent of these new products were for biotechnology drugs, indicating that a new cycle of drug development may be beginning.[1] In addition to an increased number of new products, the number of suppliers for older drugs has markedly increased. In some drug categories, the number of new suppliers for existing drugs has risen at least ten percent annually since 1982.[1]

One reason for the increases observed in new drug product introductions and the number of suppliers for older drugs is the Drug Price Competition and Patent Term Restoration Act of 1984. Research-based pharmaceutical manufacturers have increased the efficiency of their research operations and are increasing their investment into research and development because of the added patent life protection afforded by the Drug Price Competition and Patent Term Restoration Act. Generic drug suppliers are proliferating because this Act allowed companies to use abbreviated new drug application procedures to obtain product approval and because more brand name drugs will lose their patents between 1990 and 1995.

The growth in the number of generic drug suppliers and the increased introduction of new chemical entities in the pharmaceutical marketplace have not gone unnoticed by purchasers of pharmaceutical products. Corporate benefit managers and public healthcare program administrators realize that the marketplace for pharmaceuticals is changing and that the market for pharmaceuticals is becoming competitive; they are adopting a business attitude to managing their programs. Health maintenance organizations (HMOs) and preferred provider organizations have formed to serve this market, and a new term, managed health-care, has entered the jargon of health and drug industry executives.

Sandwiched between pharmaceutical manufacturers, generic drug suppliers, insurance programs, and Medicaid/Medicare are the individuals on HMO and hospital pharmacy and therapeutics (P&T) committees who must decide which drugs to place on a formulary and which supplier will be the source of these products. Their tasks become increasingly complicated as they wrestle with the problem of trying to contain costs while ensuring that quality products are purchased.

In summary, the number of new drugs and the number of suppliers of older drug products significantly increased in the 1980s. These changes occurred simultaneously with an increased emphasis by corporate purchasers and public healthcare program administrators on cost-containment procedures. The increase in the number of suppliers and drug products coupled with an emphasis on cost containment in public and private healthcare programs is creating difficult problems for decision makers who must select the most cost-effective drugs and suppliers for each therapeutic category.

Purpose and Objectives

The primary purpose of this chapter is to describe the trends in the U.S. prescription and nonprescription drug markets in terms of sales, therapeutic categories, suppliers, and other variables affecting drug usage and costs. The principal objective of this chapter is to examine drug usage within the U.S. population to determine if usage, the number of products available, and the number of suppliers are changing. Finally, this chapter discusses the implications of pharmaceutical marketplace trends on the work of P&T committee decision-makers involved in the important task of selecting cost-effective drug products.

This chapter is divided into three sections. The first section examines trends in prescription drug costs, expenditures, sales, and usage, and reasons and rationale affecting the increase or decrease in prescription drug costs, expenditures, sales, and usage. The purpose of the second section is to determine the consequences of the changes in drug use on the future behaviors of prescription drug purchasers. The last section discusses drug selection and formulary management.

Trends in the Economics and Usage of Pharmaceutical Products

EXPENDITURES AND COSTS OF PHARMACEUTICAL PRODUCTS

Drugs as a percentage of the total expenditures for personal healthcare in the U.S. have declined, as the data in Table 1 show, from a high of 9.8 percent

**Table 1. Distribution of Selected Expenditures as a Percentage of
Total Personal Healthcare, 1980–88[2]**

Year	Hospital Care (%)	Physician Services (%)	Drugs and Other Nondurable Medical Sundries (%)
1980	46.2	21.3	8.6
1981	46.8	21.5	8.1
1982	47.2	21.6	7.3
1983	46.6	21.7	7.8
1984	45.7	22.1	7.8
1985	45.0	22.3	7.7
1986	44.5	22.8	7.6
1987	39.6	19.0	7.9
1988	39.2	19.5	7.8

in 1976 to 7.0 percent in 1987.[2] Examined from a different viewpoint, the percentage change in annual expenditures for drugs and medical sundries (including dispensing fees) declined from a high of 10.6 percent in 1983 to 8.9 percent in 1987 (Table 2).[2] These patterns indicate that dollar outlays for other components of health expenditures have increased significantly while dollar outlays for pharmaceuticals have not. Possible explanations for the decline in drug costs as a percent of total health expenditures include: (1) increases in the outlay for other healthcare services, e.g., physician services, have significantly increased; and (2) the cost-containment measures implemented by third-party payers are reducing drug costs in public and private healthcare programs. Although the outlays for drugs are up, they have not increased as much as for hospital or physician services.

When one examines the percentage of change in the retail costs of prescription drugs, however, one observes, as seen in Table 3,[3,4] that the percentage change in costs for drugs is significantly higher than it is for hospital rooms and physician services.[2] Thus, while total dollar outlays for pharmaceuticals have not increased as much as the outlays for hospital rooms and physician services, the percentage change in drug prices is occurring at a higher rate.

Costs for pharmaceuticals at the retail level have increased because of the significant increase in costs of pharmaceuticals from pharmaceutical companies. The probable explanations for the increase in costs at the manufacturer level since 1982 are an increase in the investment of funds by brand manufacturers into research and development, the patent expiration of top revenue-generating products, the strength of the dollar overseas, and the increased penetration of the market for multisource products by generic drug manufacturing companies (unpublished communication, Osterhaus JT, Zellman WN, Gagnon JP. Policy and pricing: product group price changes in selected therapeutic categories, 1981–1985). Whether prices will continue to increase at a rate of nine percent in the future cannot be determined. It is conceivable that the price increases observed over the last nine years are adjustments made by pharmaceutical companies in response to impending patent losses on high-volume products. These companies need time to market new products. It is becoming increasingly difficult to identify and receive FDA approval for new chemical entities.

━━━ DRUG USE TRENDS

A logical place to begin an investigation of drug usage trends in the U.S. would be to examine how many prescriptions are dispensed annually. An examination of the data in Table 4[5] discloses that 1.54 billion prescriptions were dispensed in 1989, an increase of one percent over 1988.[6] Prescription volume in the U.S. has increased one to two percent a year over the last five years. The apparent small annual increases in retail prescriptions do not reflect the fact that the average prescription size is about 14 percent larger than it was in 1976. Baum et al. noted that "the number of prescriptions and the size of the U.S. population

Table 2. Percentage Change in Selected Expenditures on Personal Healthcare, 1980–88[2]

Year	Hospital Care (%)	Physician Services (%)	Drugs and Medical Sundries (%)
1980	16.8	16.4	9.5
1981	17.2	16.9	10.4
1982	13.5	12.8	6.9
1983	8.6	10.7	10.6
1984	6.5	10.1	8.4
1985	7.0	9.9	8.3
1986	7.4	11.1	6.6
1987	8.0	13.3	8.4
1988	9.3	13.0	8.6

Table 3. Percentage Change in Medical Care Consumer Price Index for Selected Items[3,4]

Year	Hospital Rooms (%)	Physician Services (%)	Prescription Drugs (%)	OTC Drugs (%)
1981	14.8	11.0	11.4	12
1982	15.7	9.4	11.7	11
1983	11.3	7.7	10.9	8
1984	8.3	7.0	9.6	6
1985	5.9	5.8	9.5	5
1986	6.0	7.2	8.6	
1987	7.2	7.3	8.0	
1988	9.3	7.2	8.0	

OTC = over the counter.

both increased by 16 percent from 1971 to 1985, while prescription size (i.e., doses per container) increased by 29 percent."[7] They estimate that population exposure, calculated as the number of prescriptions times the average prescription size divided by population size, indicates that outpatient drug exposure increased by 29 percent from 1971 to 1984.[7] In addition to presenting increases in prescription volume, the data in Table 4 reveal there has been a slight change in the pattern of new and refill prescriptions. The number of refill prescriptions have declined over the last two years.

Increases in prescription volume coupled with increases in prescription size indicate that the pharmaceutical market is growing. It is probable that, because of current and future changes, the pharmaceutical marketplace will grow even more over the next ten years.

DRUG PURCHASE TRENDS

IMS America, Ltd. reports annually on the purchase of pharmaceuticals by retail pharmacies and hospitals in U.S. markets. In 1989, annual purchases rose 14 percent over 1988 to $37.3 billion. An examination of the data in Table 5 reveals that the greatest percentage change in dollar purchases occurred in 1983 and that it has stabilized at ten percent a year over the last two years.[5]

Table 4. Prescriptions Dispensed in Retail Pharmacies[5]

Year	New Prescriptions	Percent Change	Refill Prescriptions	Percent Change	Total Prescriptions	Percent Change
1982	768 189 000	4.1	729 994 000	7.1	1 498 183 000	5.5
1983	742 399 000	−3.4	765 735 000	4.9	1 508 134 000	0.7
1984	750 118 000	1.0	781 630 000	2.1	1 531 748 000	1.6
1985	755 468 000	0.7	792 944 000	1.4	1 548 412 000	1.1
1986	784 483 000	3.8	773 028 000	−2.5	1 557 511 000	0.6
1987	838 560 000	4.0	774 485 000	−1.0	1 611 025 000	1.0
1988	865 657 000	3.2	765 450 000	1.2	1 631 107 000	1.3

Table 5. U.S. Pharmaceutical Market Community Pharmacies' and Hospitals' Pharmaceutical Purchases[5]

Year	Purchases ($ millions)	Percent Change
1980	12 207.2	+ 13
1981	13 758.7	+ 13
1982	15 557.9	+ 13
1983	18 158.6	+ 17
1984	20 610.3	+ 14
1985	22 711.3	+ 10
1986	25 152.7	+ 11
1987	28 843.7	+ 15
1988	33 110.9	+ 15

Pharmaceutical purchase data can be further cross-tabulated by the type of purchases, prescription or over-the-counter (OTC) drugs; and type of market, community or hospital. The data in Table 6 provide a breakdown of pharmaceutical purchases in community pharmacies. A perusal of community pharmacy drug purchases reveals that the percentage change in dollar purchases follows the same pattern as that in Table 5, except that the changes are at a higher level. The annual percentage change in hospital purchases is at an even higher level, as Table 7 shows, but has declined since 1983.[5]

Pharmaceutical purchases in community pharmacies and hospitals are increasing at a declining rate for a number of reasons. First and foremost are the cost-containment measures utilized by private and public third-party payers. Since 1982, federal and state government agencies and corporations have emphasized the need to reduce healthcare-related costs. The federal government has played a significant role in developing cost-containment measures for prescription drugs through its Medicaid program. This program, jointly administered by

Table 6. U.S. Pharmaceutical Market Retail Pharmacies' Pharmaceutical Purchases[5]

Year	Total Prescription Drug Purchases ($ millions)	Percent Change	Total OTC Drug Purchases ($ millions)	Percent Change	Total Market	Percent Change
1981	7 402.9	13.6	3 813.4	6.8	11 216.3	11.0
1982	8 567.2	15.7	3 966.1	4.0	12 533.3	12.0
1983	10 110.6	18.0	4 476.7	12.9	14 587.3	16.0
1984	11 747.7	16.2	4 798.4	7.2	16 546.1	13.0
1985	13 435.3	14.4	4 969.2	3.6	18 404.5	11.0
1986	15 146.5	12.7	5 099.2	2.6	20 245.7	10.0
1987	17 010.0	12.3	5 520.0	8.3	22 530.0	11.3
1988	21 000.0	19.0	6 000.0	8.0	27 000.0	19.8

OTC = over the counter.

Table 7. U.S. Pharmaceutical Market Hospitals' Pharmaceutical Purchases[5]

Year	Purchases ($ millions)	Percent Change
1980	2 119.2	+ 16
1981	2 539.4	+ 20
1982	3 027.5	+ 19
1983	3 572.0	+ 18
1984	4 064.2	+ 14
1985	4 296.0	+ 5
1986	4 907.0	+ 14
1987	5 572.5	+ 14
1988	6 100.7	+ 10

Table 8. Population Trends for Selected Countries

Country	Total Population (millions)		Over-60 Population (millions)		Over 60 (%)	
	1985	2020	1985	2020	1985	2020
Belgium	9 880	9 854	1 894	3 136	19	32
Netherlands	14 506	14 766	2 430	4 179	17	28
France	54 608	58 358	9 685	14 372	18	25
Germany	61 106	55 038	11 981	15 657	20	28
Italy	56 874	57 292	10 699	14 368	19	25
United Kingdom	55 640	56 398	11 309	13 331	20	24
United States	237 660	305 085	38 286	67 147	16	22
Canada	25 605	33 621	3 573	7 723	14	23
Japan	120 072	128 586	17 248	34 133	14	27

the states and the federal government, has been a proving and evaluation ground for prescription drug cost-containment techniques. States are free to experiment with various cost-containment measures by using waivers or the granting process. A number of cost-control measures have evolved out of state Medicaid programs that have been carried over to private third-party prescription plans.

The emphasis of these controls has been on drug products and pharmacy services. Included among the cost-containment measures for products have been limits on the number of prescriptions filled per month, number of prescriptions refilled per month, number of different drugs, limits on drug quantities, and on the use of brand name drugs. Other controls include the use of generic drugs, direct manufacturer cost reimbursement, quantity discounts, drug volume purchase plans, formularies, and therapeutic substitution. Pharmacy services have been controlled by using fixed-fee reimbursement, and product-only reimbursement.

INFLUENCE OF AGE ON DRUG USAGE

The most important demographic variable influencing the future growth of pharmaceutical purchases and drug usage is the growth in the number of elderly people in developed countries. The proportion of elderly in 1985 and the year 2020 for ten developed countries is presented in Table 8. An inspection of the last two columns of this table reveals that in most of these countries the proportion of their populations over 60 will almost double. This demographic trend is important to pharmaceutical companies and distributors because this age cohort consumes most of the drugs manufactured and dispensed.

Catastrophic prescription drug coverage for Medicare recipients almost became a reality. Although currently it is a moot question, it is still unclear as to what would be the cost of an outpatient drug program for the elderly. *Health Care Financing Review* recently published an article that examined this question. One of the first steps in assessing the cost of a catastrophic drug benefit for elderly citizens was to determine the prescription drug utilization rate among this age cohort if coverage was available. Using drug utilization data from a number of sources, Waldo projected past and future drug use rates among the Medicare enrollees. The average number of prescriptions per capita for 1988 was estimated to be 18.1 (Table 9).[8] This figure will rise to 19 over the next few years. Multiplying this estimate times the estimated increase in the number of elderly over 62 who will be living in the year 2000 (8 million) means that the demand for prescriptions during this time period will increase by at least 10 percent.

MAJOR THERAPEUTIC CLASSES AND DRUG CATEGORIES

The ratings of the major drug categories have not changed over the last five years (Table 10). More prescriptions are written for cardiovascular agents and systemic antiinfectives than for any other category. The categories that have experienced high growth are bronchial therapy, dermatologics, antidiabetics, antiarthritics, and antispasmodics.[6] This prescription drug use pattern differs significantly from that of OTC drug use, as seen in Table 11 (personal communication, Jones HR, Vice President, Manager, Marketing Research Group, USA HBA/Drug Industry Services, A.C. Nielsen Company, Northbrook, IL, 1987). The top OTC categories are analgesics and digestives, and cold, cough, and flu preparations. Table 11 also indicates the growth trends in units and dollars.

The growth in the number of prescriptions dispensed within drug categories reflects the changes previously discussed in the age profile of the population. Most of the top categories of drugs are those used for chronic conditions. Figure 1 shows how the share of total prescriptions for chronic therapy has grown from 57.3 percent in 1975 to 69.2 percent in 1982.

GROWTH IN NEW CHEMICAL ENTITIES

Another phenomenon fueling the use of prescription drugs has been the productivity of the U.S. pharmaceutical industry. Since 1981, the number of new chemical entities approved by the FDA has been in the double digits. The double-digit average over the last nine years was 23, with a high of 30 in 1985 (Table 12).[9] Increased efficiency in research and development by the pharmaceutical industry has positively affected the growth in outpatient prescriptions and drug purchases, because when new pharmaceuticals with significant improvements are released, physicians and patients are willing to use them. Moreover, if they are truly effective and have minimal adverse effects, they will continue to be taken and usage will significantly increase. This scenario has occurred with a number of recent ethical pharmaceutical products.

IMPACT OF FEDERAL GOVERNMENT ON PHARMACEUTICAL SALES

The activities of Congressional committees and subcommittees and administrative agencies also have affected the availability of drugs and drug usage rates.

Table 9. Medicare Enrollee Prescriptions per Capita by Age, Institutional Status, and Disability Status, 1967–91[8]

Category	1967	1973	1977	1985	1986	1987	1988	1989	1990	1991
All enrollees	10.4	13.6	14.7	17.1	17.4	17.8	18.1	18.3	18.7	19.1
Aged	10.4	13.4	14.4	16.8	17.1	17.4	17.7	18.0	18.4	18.7
institutionalized	19.8	25.5	27.3	31.3	31.8	32.4	32.9	33.5	34.1	34.7
noninstitutionalized	9.9	12.8	13.7	16.0	16.3	16.5	16.8	17.1	17.5	17.8
65–69 y	8.2	10.6	11.4	13.1	13.4	13.6	13.9	14.1	14.4	14.7
70–74 y	9.9	12.8	13.7	15.8	16.1	16.3	16.6	16.9	17.2	17.5
75–79 y	12.3	15.9	17.0	19.7	20.0	20.3	20.7	21.0	21.4	21.8
≥ 80 y	10.9	14.0	15.0	17.4	17.7	18.1	18.4	18.7	19.0	19.3
Disabled		16.5	17.7	20.5	20.9	21.3	21.7	22.0	22.5	22.9

Agencies, such as the Health Care Financing Administration (HCFA), and committees, such as the House Energy and Commerce and the Senate Labor and Human Resources Health Subcommittees, have implemented regulations and statutes that have a direct bearing on the use and sales of drugs.

The primary public healthcare programs are Medicaid and Medicare. Medicaid was a $48.7 billion program in 1988. It is projected that expenditures in this program will grow at a rate of 11 percent per year over the next three years. There are presently 22.3 million enrollees in this program, 15.3 million of which are prescription drug users. The total amount of money expended on prescription drugs in 1988 was $3.2 million.[10]

Medicare was a $76 billion program in 1986 that is projected to grow at a rate of 9 percent over the next three years. There are over 31 million recipients of Medicare benefits in the U.S. Approximately two-thirds of the payments in

Table 10. Major Therapeutic Classes and Drug Categories, 1988[6]

Rank	Drug Class	Total Prescriptions (millions)	Percent Total Prescriptions	Percent Change
1	Cardiovascular	242	15	−1
2	Systemic antiinfectives	217	13	3
3	Psychotherapeutics	139	8	−1
4	Ethical analgesics	117	7	1
5	Diuretics	91	6	−8
6	Hormones	91	6	5
7	Antiarthritics	79	5	2
8	Antispasmatics and GI/GU	61	4	5
9	Cough and cold preparations	24	1	9
10	Contraceptives	58	4	−2
11	Bronchial therapy	66	4	5
12	Dermatologics	49	3	12
13*	Ophthalmic preparations	38	2	2
14*	Nutrients and supplements	37	2	−1
15	Diabetes	39	2	2
16	Ethical sedatives	28	2	−5

*Not listed in 1988.
GI = gastrointestinal; GU = genitourinary.

Table 11. Over-the-Counter Sales by Use

Total OTCs	1985 ($ millions)	Average Annual Percentage Change	
		$	Units
Cold/cough/flu	6,940	9	2
Analgesics, digestives	1,870	12	3
Other internal medications	4,300	8	1
Externally used medications	770	8	4

OTCs = over-the-counter sales.

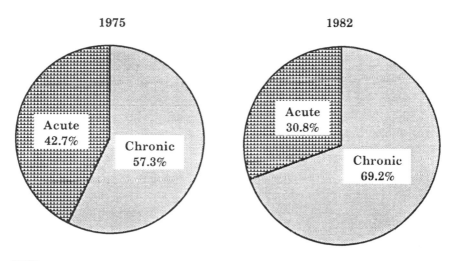

1975   1982

Figure 1. Share of total prescriptions for acute versus chronic therapy.

Table 12. New Chemical Entities Approved, 1981–89[9]

1981	1982	1983	1984	1985	1986	1987	1988	1989
27	28	14	22	30	20	21	20	23

this program are for hospital services and one-third for physician services. Only inpatient hospital prescription drugs are currently covered under Medicare but, as was previously mentioned, Congress attempted to implement a law that was to offer catastrophic coverage for outpatient prescription drugs for Medicare recipients. It was expected that coverage of outpatient prescription drugs by public and private third-party payers would have increased from approximately 30 percent to over 40 percent.[10] It is not clear whether the Department of Health and Human Services (DHHS) will continue the study to evaluate potential methods to improve drug utilization review activities for covered drugs. In addition, the DHHS needs to pursue a longitudinal study that assesses the use of covered outpatient prescription drugs by Medicare beneficiaries. Components of the study should include an assessment of a drug's medical necessity, the potential for adverse drug reactions, a drug cost evaluation, and an evaluation of a patient's stockpiling and wasting of medication.

Outpatient prescription coverage by public and private third-party programs influences drug usage. Drug usage among enrollees in these programs usually increases because drugs are available without cost to the patient. However, these programs usually contain cost-containment measures designed to reduce drug costs, e.g., the HCFA through its strong support of the use of generic drugs in state Medicaid programs has promoted the growth of the generic drug industry.

Table 13. Number of Suppliers for Products in the Most-Prescribed Drug Categories, 1983–87*

Drug Category	1983		1984		1985		1986		1987	
	n	% change	n	% change	n	% change	n	% change	n	% change
Analgesics	79	–10.2	83	5.1	88	6.0	95	8.0	110	15.8
Antiarthritics	266	–0.4	297	11.7	338	13.8	389	15.1	515	32.4
Antibiotics	497	6.9	636	28.0	724	13.8	728	0.6	850	16.8
Antihypertensives	395	15.8	379	4.1	421	11.1	474	12.6	569	20.0
Beta-blockers	5	0.0	7	40.0	8	14.3	29	262.5	46	58.6
Bronchodilators	231	2.7	156	–32.5	172	10.3	224	30.2	272	21.4
Diuretics	329	29.5	347	5.5	397	14.4	352	–11.3	399	13.4
Oral contraceptives	15	0.0	15	0.0	15	0.0	15	0.0	16	6.7
Tranquilizers	70	22.8	114	62.9	158	38.6	159	0.6	214	34.6
Vasodilators	270	–1.5	316	17.0	290	–8.2	323	11.4	359	11.2

*The total number of suppliers in each category is not unique. If a supplier provided two different drugs in a category, it was counted twice in this analysis.

Table 14. Product Trend Data for the Most-Prescribed Drug Categories, 1983–87

Drug Category	1983		1984		1985		1986		1987	
	n	% change	n	% change	n	% change	n	% change	n	% change
Analgesics	11	0.0	15	36.4	16	6.7	19	18.8	17	10.5
Antiarthritics	34	13.3	26	–23.5	26	0.0	30	15.4	30	0.0
Antihypertensives	41	10.8	39	–4.9	41	5.1	41	0.0	42	2.4
Beta-blockers	5	0.0	7	40.0	8	14.3	29	262.5	46	58.6
Bronchodilators	20	–4.8	13	–35.0	13	0.0	16	23.1	16	0.0
Diuretics	24	9.1	24	0.0	26	8.3	25	–3.9	25	0.0
Oral contraceptives	10	0.0	10	0.0	10	0.0	10	0.0	10	0.0
Tranquilizers	15	0.0	18	2.0	17	5.6	16	5.9	17	6.3
Vasodilators	8	0.0	12	50.0	11	8.3	14	27.3	14	0.0

Through passage of the Drug Price Competition and Patent Term Restoration Act in 1984, the House and Senate Health Subcommittees assisted the growth of generic companies but also gave significant incentives to research-based pharmaceutical companies to conduct research. The net effect of this bill has been to increase the number of suppliers for each class of drugs. The percentage change in the number of suppliers for drugs in the top drug categories has been growing at an increasing rate for half of the top drug categories over the last five years (Table 13). While the number of drug products in the top drug categories have increased over the last five years (Table 14), the percentage change has not been as dramatic as it is for the number of suppliers and has been significant only for beta-blockers. It is obvious from scanning the data in these two tables that the 1984 Drug Price Competition and Patent Term Restoration Act has had the immediate effect of stimulating competition for drugs off patent.

Consequence of the Changes in Drug Use

The net effect of the changes just discussed will have significant impact on all sectors of healthcare and providers. Prescription usage could significantly increase over the next ten years. Community and hospital pharmacists will have a large choice of drug suppliers from which to select products. The variety of suppliers creates difficult problems for P&T committees because they must decide which suppliers will be available on the hospital's formulary.

Whether significant breakthrough drugs will be developed is still open for debate. It is quite evident that the research-based companies are investing significant funds into research and development (Table 15). In 1989, these companies invested $5.6 billion in domestic research and development, an increase of 11.8 percent. It is conceivable that this level of investment could produce significant numbers of breakthrough drugs over the next decade.

The work of P&T committees will become more complex because of the changes that are occurring. At the present time, many drug product decisions are handled by P&T committees during monthly meetings. A staff of pharmacists and technicians will conduct computer-assisted analyses of proposed drugs for these committees in the future because of the number of suppliers and the complexity of the drugs. P&T committees presently are composed mostly of physi-

Table 15. Domestic Research and Development Expenditures for Human-Use Ethical Pharmaceuticals, 1982–86[11]

	1982	1983	1984	1985	1986
Expenditure ($ millions)	2 265.6	2 663.1	2 976.4	3 370.7	3 813.3*
Percent change		17.6	11.8	13.3	13.1

*Budgeted.

cians who do not have the expertise to select a drug product supplier. In the future, pharmacists will select suppliers using objective data obtained through surveys. Factors such as product quality, product information, economics, service quality, and company reputation will be used to contrast and compare companies. Cues (e.g., returns policy, bioequivalence data) that allow pharmacists to objectively measure a factor will have to be identified. Moreover, pharmacists will have to be trained to use factors and cues in evaluating companies. There is little doubt that as more pharmacists become computer literate, the process of selecting a drug for a formulary as well as a manufacturer will become more objective.

Course of Action for Product Selection

Individuals involved in product selection, whether it be for a formulary or a prescription, must be taught to consider a number of variables in addition to product cost. William Roper, in the fall of 1987, noted that Medicaid had entered its third decade. The focus of the program during the first decade was accessibility, i.e., making sure that everyone eligible for Medicaid was able to access the program. During the second decade of Medicaid's existence the emphasis was on cost containment, e.g., the maximum allowable cost regulations and generic dispensing to lower program costs. Over the next decade, according to Roper, Medicaid will underscore the need to maintain quality.[12] The objective of pharmacists involved in product selection for formularies should be to identify the highest quality product for the most economic price. Cost has been easy to use because it can be objectively measured. Other attributes, such as adverse effects and quality of life, will have to be factored into future decisions to select a product for a formulary.

Summary

The purpose of this chapter was to describe and discuss the U.S. prescription and nonprescription drug markets in terms of cost, drug usage, therapeutic categories, and other variables. Its primary objective was to show that in the future, drug use will increase because of changes in the age groups of the population and the increased efficiency and level of investment of the pharmaceutical industry in research and development. It also showed that the number of suppliers of multisource products will continue to accelerate. The net effect of these changes on community and hospital pharmacies, formulary decision-makers, and physicians will be the increased difficulty of selecting a pharmaceutical product for a given illness and a supplier for the product. Subsequent chapters will address the methodologies and approaches that decision-makers can implement to make the increasingly difficult task of selecting manufacturers and drug products more objective.

References

1. Prescription drug sales soar in year of ferment. *Drug Store News* 1987;9(9):135-8.

2. U.S. Health Care Financing Administration, Division of National Cost Estimates, Washington, DC, 1987.

3. U.S. Bureau of Labor Statistics, Washington, DC, 1988.

4. Business Economics Department, Metropolitan Life Insurance Company, 1987.

5. National prescription audit. IMS America, Ltd., Ambler, PA.

6. Prescription drug market confirms upward trend. *Drug Topics* 1990;*134*:52-4, 57-8, 60.

7. Baum C, Kennedy DL, Knapp DE, Faich GA. Drug utilization in the U.S.—1985: seventh annual review. U.S. Food and Drug Administration, U.S. Dept. of Commerce, National Technical Information Service (PB87-149902), Rockville, MD, Dec. 1986.

8. Waldo DR. Outpatient prescription drug spending by the Medicare population. *Health Care Financ Rev* 1987;9(1):83-9.

9. FDA approval and drug introductions compiled. *Med Market Media* 1990;*25*(4):42.

10. Pharmaceutical benefits state and medical programs. Washington, DC: National Pharmaceutical Council, 1989:86-7.

11. 1987–1989 Annual survey report. Washington, DC: Pharmaceutical Manufacturers Association, 1989:19.

12. Robert Woods Johnson health policy. Fellows meeting. Washington, DC, October 1988.

3

Cost Determination and Analysis

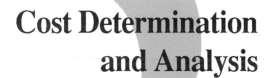

Lon N. Larson

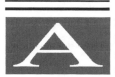ny program and activity, including drug therapy, consumes resources and produces consequences. The resources consumed are its costs. Economists also calculate the resources consumed by a disease; this is referred to as cost of illness.

The cost of an illness is the sum of three components: (1) direct medical costs, (2) direct nonmedical costs, and (3) indirect costs. Included among direct medical costs are the amount spent on medical services to treat the illness, including hospital care, professional services, drugs, and supplies. Direct nonmedical costs are out-of-pocket expenses for items outside the medical-care sector. For instance, transportation to the site of treatment, lodging for the family during treatment, and hiring help for the home are direct expenses for nonmedical services. Nonetheless, these are part of the cost of illness. Finally, indirect costs are the earnings lost as a result of temporary or permanent disability occurring because of the illness. Unpaid family assistance in the home is another indirect cost. The concept of indirect costs is derived from the human capital approach of valuing life.

Please note that economist and accountant have different definitions of the term indirect costs. The economic view was presented above. In accounting, indirect costs are overhead expenses related to the production of several products.

The costs of medical programs or treatments can fit into the same classification. To illustrate with a simplified example, chronic renal dialysis may be done at clinics or at home. Clinic dialysis entails more direct medical care costs because special facilities and medical personnel are involved. Travel expense to the facility is a direct nonmedical expense. Finally, if the patient must miss work, the lost wages are an indirect cost. In comparison, home dialysis also includes equipment and supplies (direct medical costs). Facility fees and transportation costs are less important; however, home dialysis requires a trained helper. The helper's time (whether paid or not) is a cost of the treatment. A comparison of these dialysis alternatives must include all of these costs.

Extending this example to a comparison of the costs and benefits of chronic dialysis, the benefits of the treatment include a reduction in the cost of endstage renal disease. As death is averted, the lost earnings associated with premature mortality are reduced. Likewise, the medical costs incurred for palliative care prior to death from endstage renal disease are also saved through dialysis. However, other medical costs arise because dialysis prolongs life. The costs of treating cancer, pneumonia, anxiety, and so on, that are acquired in the additional years of life are included as a cost of dialysis.

The economic effects of a medical care treatment may be viewed as the sum of its costs and benefits. The costs include: (1) the cost of the treatment itself, (2) the cost of treating adverse effects, and (3) the medical costs incurred during extended life-years (if mortality is postponed). These are the direct, medical costs of treatment. Two other costs may also be involved: (4) expenses incurred for nonmedical services (e.g., transportation), and (5) earnings lost by the patient or family members as a result of receiving the treatment (i.e., indirect costs). The benefits of the treatment relate to its impact on the costs of illness. The items are similar conceptually to those above and include the medical costs, nonmedical expenses, and lost earnings associated with the illness that are avoided or saved because of the treatment.

This chapter concentrates on direct medical care costs, which often are the most important in assessing the costs of alternative medical treatments. The chapter is divided into four sections. The first is an explanation of opportunity cost, which is the economic basis for valuing resource consumption. The second section provides a framework for determining the costs of a program or service. This framework encompasses four components: (1) determining the scope of costs to be included, (2) specifying the "ingredients" or inputs, (3) assigning dollar values to the ingredients, and (4) allowing for uncertainty. In the third part of the chapter, topics related to assigning dollar values are discussed. These topics include market prices, the relationship between costs and output levels, differences in timing, valuing capital projects, and the allocation of shared costs. The final part of this chapter deals with the costs of items frequently included in pharmacoeconomic evaluations. Sometimes, actual examples can help clarify a formal description of a topic as presented here. The reader may want to refer to studies cited at the end of this chapter to see how costs were handled.

Opportunity Cost—The Economist's View of Cost

The cost of a good or service is the value of the resources that are consumed in its production. For instance, treatment for a disease may consume such resources as drug products and pharmacist services, physician services, laboratory and radiology procedures, and hospital and nursing home care. These services, in turn, are intermediate goods whose production requires the basic resources of personnel, equipment and supplies, and facilities. Thus, the cost of treatment is the value of the intermediate services consumed, and the cost of each intermediate service is the value of the basic resources that it consumes.

For the economist, the value of a resource is its opportunity cost, which may be defined as "the amount that an input could earn in its best alternative use, or the alternative that must be foregone when something is produced."[1] The opportunity cost is what could have been produced with the same resources; that is, the value of the alternative foregone.

An example may help clarify the concept of opportunity cost. Tertiary and primary services frequently are compared in health policy discussions, where the cost of a tertiary service (e.g., organ transplant) is expressed in terms of the primary care services (e.g., perinatal services) that could be purchased with the same sum of dollars. In essence, this is a statement about the opportunity cost of tertiary care. That is, primary care is assumed to be the alternative that is foregone when tertiary care is produced, and the unrealized benefits of primary care become the opportunity cost of the tertiary service.

A Framework for Determining Costs [2,3]

DETERMINING THE SCOPE

In determining the costs of a program or treatment, the first step is to decide from whose perspective the analysis is to be undertaken. Economic evaluations may assume the viewpoint of a single provider, insurer, the healthcare system, or society. An example will help clarify this point.

Consider a Medicare patient as she moves through the various levels of care from hospital, to an extended-care facility, to home. In the hospital's view, its relevant costs are those incurred during the hospital stay. For instance, the hospital welcomes drug therapy that can reduce the length of stay and/or other services during the stay. An earlier discharge, however, may mean that more intensive and more costly nursing home care are required. This is relevant from the perspectives of the healthcare system and Medicare; it is irrelevant to the hospital.

Finally, when the patient is transferred to her home, a family member assumes the role of care-giver. From society's perspective, the care-giver's time is a cost; however, the cost is outside the realm of the healthcare system and outside the coverage of Medicare.

Thus, the cost of a healthcare program depends on one's perspective. An initial step in determining costs is to specify the perspective of the study and, thereby, delineate the scope of relevant costs.

====== SPECIFYING THE INGREDIENTS

A second step in cost determination is to identify the resources consumed by the program; that is, the "ingredients."[4] Identifying ingredients precedes assigning values to them, even though the two steps often are done simultaneously.

The goal is to identify and specify all resources consumed in conjunction with a program or treatment. With healthcare programs, it can be helpful to separate resources into two types: basic resources and intermediate services. The former are used in the production of the latter, which are used in producing treatments. Examples of each are outlined in Table 1.

If one were interested in determining the cost of a pharmacy service, the focus would be on the basic resources consumed in its production (e.g., pharmacist time, other personnel time, drug product costs, and other supplies). If, on the other hand, the issue was the cost of treating a disease, the focus may shift to the intermediate services (e.g., hospital, laboratory, and pharmacy services). Some evaluations will look at both basic resources and intermediate services. In comparing the cost of two drug regimens, for instance, basic resources may be used in the analysis of the pharmacy component, while intermediate services are used for the other components.

A key point is that to be meaningful, an economic evaluation must include all relevant resources, and not just the ones that are obvious and/or easy to identify and measure. The ingredients approach of identifying the inputs separately from assigning a dollar value to them is a means of reducing the likelihood of overlooking relevant items.

====== ASSIGNING DOLLAR VALUES

Once the resources used in a program have been identified, these inputs are assigned a monetary value. This is often quite complex. As a general rule, the time and effort spent in assigning a monetary value should be proportional to the

Table 1. Common Ingredients

Basic Resources	Intermediate Services
Personnel	Pharmaceutical services
professional	Physician services
administrative	medical/visits
support	surgical
Equipment and supplies	Laboratory tests
drug products	Hospital services
supplies (e.g., vials, administration sets)	inpatient
Facilities	ancillary services
	room and board (hotel) services
	outpatient
	Other

importance of that resource. Major resources or cost items should receive more attention than minor items.

Several factors enter into this valuation process. One is the relationship between costs of production (i.e., expenses) and the volume of output. Since not all expenses vary proportionately with output, distinctions must be made between average and marginal costs. A second factor is that some resources may be shared among several activities or programs and, therefore, must be allocated. A third factor is that not all costs may be incurred at the same time; future costs must be discounted so as to be comparable to current costs. These issues are addressed in the next part of this chapter.

ALLOWING FOR UNCERTAINTY

Costs often are not known with certainty; assumptions are made and estimated figures are derived. A method to compensate for this uncertainty is sensitivity analysis, in which the economic evaluation is reworked using different assumptions or estimates of the uncertain costs.

Sensitivity analysis can be viewed as a "what if" analysis: What if a price increase (decrease) for a drug product is assumed? What if a different hospital per diem is used? What if different manpower requirements are assumed? Again, sensitivity analysis is essential for any cost that is not known with certainty. To assume that assumptions and estimates are factual can lead to erroneous conclusions.

Value Assigned to Ingredients

This section concerns the issues involved in assigning monetary values to resources: (1) market prices, (2) relationship between costs and output volume, (3) time differences and discounting, and (4) shared costs and cost allocation.

MARKET PRICES

Although opportunity cost is the true cost of consuming a resource, market prices are probably the best indicator of value and should be used when available.[2] For instance, market prices are appropriate for salaries and wages, equipment expenses, and drug products. Among intermediate services, market prices can be used for services rendered by outpatient laboratories, physicians, community pharmacists, and outpatient treatment centers. Third-party payment schedules can be used as an indicator of market prices. This is appropriate if the schedule is similar to actual charges and is not artificially low.

For some health services, however, market prices may not be appropriate. Hospital charges, for instance, can be misleading, because they may bear little (if any) relationship to costs. If market prices are not appropriate, values must be derived from financial records or cost accounting data.

RELATIONSHIP BETWEEN COST AND
OUTPUT VOLUME

In assigning monetary value, the relationship between cost and output volume is important. Specifically, the average cost can be deceptive, because it is not necessarily the cost of producing one more unit, nor the savings that result from producing one less unit.

Expenses (production costs) differ in behavior as output volume changes.[5] Some expenses are fixed; that is, they are unaffected by changes in output volume. Some examples are depreciation, utilities, accounting fees, insurance, interest expense, and maintenance. For a community pharmacy or hospital, these expenses remain unchanged even though the volume of output may change (i.e., numbers of prescriptions or patient days). Thus, average fixed cost (fixed cost per unit) decreases as output increases, since the fixed cost can be spread over more units.

A second category is variable expenses. As their title implies, these expenses vary with changes in the volume of output. Examples include cost of goods sold (i.e., drug product costs) and bad debts. These expenses change as the volume of activity changes; that is, the total amount spent on these items increases as volume of output increases. Average variable cost (variable cost per unit) remains virtually unchanged as volume increases or decreases.

A third category is the semi-fixed expense. Personnel expense is the principal example. Over a certain range of output levels, the expense remains unchanged. However, given sufficient changes in output, the expense increases or decreases. Some institutions have attempted to make personnel expense less fixed by using "on-call" or temporary personnel. Essentially, this reduces underutilized fixed expenses.

These expense behaviors underlie the difference between average and marginal costs. Average cost is simply total costs (fixed and variable) divided by the number of units produced. Marginal cost is the change in total cost that results from producing one additional unit of output.[1] In addition to this definition, marginal cost often is used to refer to incremental costs: the cost of one program compared with another.

In valuing the resources consumed in the production of one more unit of output, marginal cost is a better indicator than is average cost. This is because the fixed expenses, which are included in the average cost, would have been consumed, even in the absence of the additional unit. Likewise, when a unit of output is not produced (e.g., a shortened hospital stay), the amount saved is the marginal cost of the avoided output rather than its average cost. The problem is that, unlike average cost, the marginal cost is almost never known; it is not reported, nor easily derived, in accounting reports.

The importance of marginality is shown vividly by the widely cited case of the "sixth stool guaiac." As a means to detect colon cancer, the American Cancer

Society recommended up to six sequential stool guaiacs. Six was chosen because that number of tests would detect all cases (i.e., all false negatives would be caught). With this protocol, the average cost per cancer found was about $2500; however, the marginal cost per cancer found by the sixth stool guaiac was over $41 million.[6]

Distinguishing between marginal and average costs is also very important in valuing reductions in hospital length of stay. When a stay is reduced by one day, the cost savings (i.e., resources not consumed) are not the average daily cost, but rather the marginal or additional cost—including room, board, and ancillary services—associated with that day.

ADJUSTING FOR DIFFERENCES IN THE TIMING OF COSTS [7]

A time preference is associated with money. We prefer to receive dollars now rather than later, because they can generate benefits or returns in the interim. For the same reason, we prefer to pay out dollars later rather than now. In other words, a dollar today is worth more than a dollar tomorrow. As a simple example, suppose a lottery winner had the choice of receiving a million dollars today or a million dollars spread over 20 years; in all likelihood, the total sum would be taken today, so as to allow more time to enjoy and/or invest the money.

Because current and future dollars are not valued the same, future costs must be discounted to reflect their current value, when a program extends over multiple years. The present value (PV) can be calculated by multiplying the future cost (FC) by the discount factor (DF). The discount factor is dependent on two variables: the number of years into the future that the expense is incurred (n) and the discount rate (r). Thus, discounting can be expressed by the formula:

$$PV = FC \times DF(n, r) \qquad \text{Eq. 1}$$

(Mathematically, the discount factor is equal to $(1 + r)^{-n}$, where r is the discount rate, and n is the year incurred.) An abbreviated table of discount factors is shown in Table 2.

The present value of a multiyear cost stream is simply the sum of the present value of the costs for each year. An example may help. Let's assume that a hypothetical treatment regimen has costs as follows: $3000 in the first year, $2000 in the second year, and $1000 each year thereafter. Over three years, the unad-

Table 2. Discount Factors—for Calculating Present Value

n	r = 5%	r = 6%	r = 7%	r = 10%
1	0.952	0.943	0.935	0.909
2	0.907	0.890	0.873	0.826
3	0.864	0.840	0.816	0.751
4	0.823	0.792	0.763	0.683
5	0.784	0.747	0.713	0.621

justed cost is $6000. With a discount rate of 6 percent, the discount factors for costs incurred at the end of years one through three are 0.943, 0.890, and 0.840, respectively. The value of the cost stream over three years is:

$$(\$3000 \times 0.943) + (2000 \times 0.890) + (1000 \times 0.840) = \$5549 \qquad \text{Eq. 2}$$

The impact of two assumptions should be noted. In this calculation, we assumed that the expenses were incurred at the end of the period; therefore, the first year's costs (12 months in the future) were discounted using the factor for n=1, the costs for the second year (24 months out) were discounted by the factor for n=2, and so on.

An equally acceptable assumption is that the expenses are incurred at the beginning of each year. Thus, the first year's costs are current, not future, and need not be discounted. The second year's costs (12 months in the future) are discounted with the factor of n=1; for the third year (24 months) the factor of n=2 is used. In this case, the cost stream would be:

$$(\$3000 \times 1.0) + (2000 \times 0.943) + (1000 \times 0.890) = \$5776 \qquad \text{Eq. 3}$$

The second assumption relates to the discount rate. Using a higher discount rate reduces the present value of future dollars. For instance, with a 10 percent discount rate, the discount factors for ends of years one through three are 0.909, 0.826, and 0.751, respectively. In our example, this discount rate would have resulted in a present value of:

$$\$5130 = (3000 \times 0.909) + (2000 \times 0.826) + (1000 \times 0.751) \qquad \text{Eq. 4}$$

A key issue is which discount or interest rate to use; the interest rate signifies the extent or magnitude of the difference in value between a current and future dollar. As illustrated above, if they are relatively close in value, a lower discount rate is in order. As the relative value of current dollars increases, the discount rate also increases.

There is no set rule as to the best discount rate to use in economic evaluations. Theoretically, the discount rate may reflect the rate of return possible in private-sector investments, or it may reflect the social rate of time preference. The latter is society's collective time preference, as measured by the real interest rate (interest rate minus rate of inflation) on long-term government securities.

Typically, in economic evaluations, future costs do not reflect inflation; for example, if a chronic drug therapy currently costs $150 per year, that same cost is used for future years. Correspondingly, future costs are discounted by a real interest rate that excludes the effect of inflation.

In practice, sensitivity analysis is used frequently, in which a range of rates is used in the calculations. Two recommendations in selecting the range of discount rates are: government-recommended rates (5, 7, and 10 percent) and the rates used in previous studies in the area.[2]

CAPITAL PROJECTS[7]

Capital projects include plant (facilities) and equipment that have an extended (multiyear) useful life and are used in the production of other goods and services.

Typically, capital expenditures are converted into an annual expense for each year in the life of the project, discounted to reflect the time value of money. To account for both the opportunity cost of the investment (what the money could earn elsewhere) and the depreciation of the asset, the capital expenditure is annuitized. In other words, the capital expenditures are converted to the annual sum which, discounted over the life of the project, is equivalent to the capital expenditure.

This annual sum can be calculated by dividing the capital expense by the annuity factor which, like the discount factor, is based on the life expectancy and discount rate. An abbreviated table of annuity factors is shown in Table 3. As an example, a capital expenditure of $10 000 with a life span of five years and a discount rate of 6 percent yields an annualized expense of $2374; i.e., 10 000 divided by 4.212 (the annuity factor for 6 percent, n=5).

ALLOCATING SHARED COSTS[8]

Direct costs are resources consumed exclusively in the production of a single product or service. However, several costs are shared among several programs or departments; that is, they are not exclusively associated with one product or service. In accounting, these are referred to as overhead or indirect costs. Cost allocation systems are designed to distribute these overhead expenses appropriately among product lines or revenue departments (i.e., the final outputs). (Please note that in economics, the term indirect costs is used to refer to those costs that do not involve direct payments, e.g., earnings lost through morbidity.)

To illustrate, a prescription department may use some, but not all, of several expense items: rent, utilities, administration, marketing expense, and interest expense. These are indirect costs; they are used in the production of all of the firm's product lines or revenue centers.

Whether an expense is direct or indirect is situational. For instance, if advertising is for a specific product, it is a direct expense that can be charged to that

Table 3. Annuity Factors—for Calculating Present Value

n	r = 5%	r = 6%	r = 7%	r = 10%
1	0.952	0.943	0.935	0.909
2	1.859	1.833	1.808	1.736
3	2.723	2.673	2.624	2.487
4	3.546	3.465	3.387	3.170
5	4.329	4.212	4.100	3.791

particular product. However, if the advertising is for several products, the expense needs to be allocated among those products.

The details of allocation systems are beyond the scope of this chapter; however, one fundamental issue is the basis by which an overhead expense is to be allocated. Costs can be allocated on the basis of square feet, payroll, and sales, among others. For example, expenses tied to area (e.g., rent, utilities) are allocated logically on the basis of square feet; however, square feet may not be appropriate for general administrative expense and advertising, which may be better allocated using payroll and sales, respectively.

Pharmacoeconomic Applications

This part of the chapter is devoted to exploring methods of determining the costs of various services of importance in pharmaceutical-related evaluations: the cost of dispensing a prescription, personnel time, drug product costs, and hospital costs.

COST OF DISPENSING

In an outpatient pharmacy, the price charged for a prescription may be viewed as the sum of three items: (1) cost of the drug product, (2) costs of preparing the prescription, and (3) return on investment. Respectively, these three are also referred to as the cost of goods sold, the cost of dispensing, and profit.

Unless the pharmacy is exclusively a prescription shop, the costs associated with the prescription department are not equal to the expenses found on the accounting statements. Thus, the first task is to determine the sum of the expenses associated with the prescription department; the cost of dispensing then can be calculated by dividing total expenses by the number of prescriptions. Thus, determining the cost of dispensing is largely an exercise in cost allocation.

An allocation system for community pharmacies is illustrative of the principles involved. This system (which is typical of others) divides expenses into four types.[9] The first is direct expenses, which do not need to be allocated and are the expenses that can be traced to the prescription department exclusively. They include prescription-related supplies and equipment, professional fees (e.g., licensure, continuing education), professional liability insurance premiums, and expenses associated with computer systems and delivery (assuming these are prescription-only services).

The second category of expense is personnel, which is allocated on the basis of time. Each employee's salary is allocated to the prescription department based on the proportion of time spent in prescription-related activities. (To the extent that employee-related expenses can be identified with individual employees, they too can be allocated on the basis of hours; otherwise, they are a fixed cost and allocated as described below.)

The third category is indirect, fixed costs. Examples include maintenance and repairs, utilities, phone, accounting and legal fees, insurance, taxes, and interest expense. These are allocated to the prescription department on the basis of square footage; that is, the proportion of the total area devoted to the prescription department.

The fourth and final category is the indirect, variable expenses. These are allocated on the basis of sales; that is, the ratio of prescription sales to total sales. An example of an indirect, variable expense is bad debts.

PERSONNEL TIME

In the cost of dispensing discussed above, personnel expenses were allocated to the prescription department on the basis of time; that is, the proportion of hours spent in prescription-related activities. Some economic evaluations, however, require time data for specific activities. For instance, the time devoted to dosage preparation and administration may be needed in assessing drugs with different dosing schedules or in evaluating drug distribution systems.

Work measurement techniques can be used to acquire this information. Two techniques are relevant in cost determination: work sampling and stopwatch time study.[10] In work sampling, momentary observations are made at preselected times. After sufficient observations, the percentage of time devoted to each activity (including idle time) can be determined (i.e., the number of observations for an activity divided by the total number of observations). Work sampling is especially useful with nonrepetitive tasks that are not entirely uniform from occurrence to occurrence.

Stopwatch time studies, on the other hand, are useful with repetitive tasks that are of short duration. This method directly measures the time required to complete a task or activity; for instance, the time to type a label or the time to mix a solution. Again, several observations of several persons are required to derive an average time for an average worker.

After the time has been determined using these techniques, the appropriate wage rates can be applied to derive the final labor costs.

There is one cautionary note in order pertaining to opportunity cost: specifically, the opportunity cost of labor may not be reflected in the payroll. For example, if a hospital implements a new service without adding any personnel, this does not mean that the labor costs of the service are zero. Rather, the labor devoted to the program, while already on the payroll, has an opportunity cost because it could have been devoted to other activities. Thus, the market value of the labor devoted to the program is rightfully considered a cost of the program.

Similarly, a program may free some personnel time, but not affect the payroll. A notable example is administration of a once- versus three-times-daily drug in a facility. Obviously, nursing time is reduced. Although the payroll may be unaffected, time is available to devote to other opportunities.

====== DRUG PRODUCT COSTS

Drug products may have multiple prices. Buying groups, contractual agreements, quantity discounts, and competitive bidding have resulted in several prices for drug products. In economic evaluations, the appropriate price to use is the average wholesale price (AWP). Although the AWP is oftentimes higher than actual acquisition cost, it is a standard price that is available to all purchasers. Thus, findings based on AWP may be more applicable to other settings than findings based on a special contract price. Further, average wholesale prices enable more realistic comparisons between the products of different manufacturers. Again, the actual acquisition costs may be tempered by special contracts with one manufacturer, but not another.

====== HOSPITAL COSTS

Assigning value to hospital services is among the most difficult tasks in pharmaceutical-related economic evaluations, and often one of the most critical. Given their magnitude relative to other medical services, an error in valuing hospital services can easily overwhelm other costs and result in misleading conclusions. Again, a cardinal rule is the more important (i.e., larger) a cost item, the more time and effort its valuation deserves. Thus, hospital services, the most expensive of healthcare services, deserve special attention in pharmacoeconomic analyses.

The specific method of valuing hospital services depends on the nature of the study and on the data available.[2,8] The analyst's goal is to answer the questions: what resources have been used (saved) and what is their value? We will consider four options commonly available: an overall per diem cost (or charge) that encompasses all hospital services, charge data by service, ratio of costs-to-charges by service, and payment rates by diagnosis-related groups (DRGs).

An overall per diem cost (or charge) figure may be deceiving. The per diem figure is simply the average daily cost; that is, the sum of all costs (routine and all ancillaries) divided by the number of patient days. The per diem cost suffers two problems. One, it is an average of all fixed and variable costs that is not equivalent to the marginal cost. As a hospital experiences one additional (or one less) patient day, the resources consumed (saved) are equal to the marginal cost and not the average cost. Two, a per diem assumes that all days are equal in terms of resource consumption. However, the initial days of a stay are almost always more intensive in ancillary use than are the latter days.

Let us assume that one treatment alternative is associated with an average length of stay that is one day less than an alternative treatment. To use the per diem cost of the hospital (or one of its units) as the value of that day saved will likely overstate the resources actually saved.

A second, more refined option is to separate routine services from ancillary (or medical) services. Routine services are those that are relatively standard across all patient days (i.e., room, dietary, laundry, administration). For these services, the average daily cost applies to each day. (It is not equal to marginal cost, and sensitivity analysis to account for this is appropriate.) Ancillary or medical services (e.g., pharmacy, laboratory, radiology) vary by patient. Therefore, it is appropriate for these data to be collected for each patient.

Thus, in our example of valuing a one-day reduction in average length of stay, the routine services would be valued separately from ancillaries. The average daily value of routine services would be added to the value of the ancillaries consumed. The values may be charges or costs.

Typically, hospital claims data indicate the charges incurred for room and board (i.e., room rates) and the charges for each ancillary department. A potential problem with charge data is that hospital charges may not be reflective of costs (i.e., resources consumed). Some services may have higher mark-ups and subsidize other services or departments. For instance, pharmacy charges typically are relatively high compared with pharmacy costs, and room charges may be less than routine costs associated with a day in the hospital. This can pose problems for generalizing results to other hospitals because each hospital can use a different charge structure. Further, since services substituting for each other have differing mark-ups, the results of an analysis using charges may not reflect the true impact on resource consumption.

Charges can be converted to costs using cost-to-charge ratios, which vary among hospitals. These ratios typically may use allocated rather than direct costs and, consequently, include overhead expenses. A ratio is determined for each department or revenue center within the hospital. This ratio, multiplied by the charge figure from a given department, will convert that figure to its underlying cost. Cost figures avoid some of the problems of charge data mentioned above.

A final valuation is the payment rate for DRGs. This can be useful if it is indicative of actual costs and not artificially low because of political or noneconomic factors. This global payment rate is useful in valuing admissions avoided or incurred. However, if one is interested in comparing two treatment alternatives for a given DRG, the global payment rate is not very useful. For instance, if a treatment is capable of being done on an outpatient basis, the DRG payment rate may be a useful measure of the inpatient resources saved. However, in comparing two inpatient treatments for the same DRG, the payment rate is meaningless (though a cost system based on DRGs could be revealing).

In sum, one must be cautious in valuing the resources consumed (saved) in hospital services. Sensitivity analysis using various assumptions is certainly appropriate, if not essential.

Summary

This chapter has attempted to provide sufficiently detailed information to allow the reader to more critically evaluate cost analyses and possibly conduct such analyses. The reader is encouraged to critique published studies as to their methods of determining costs, by asking the following questions:

1. Are the relevant ingredients included?
2. Is each ingredient valued appropriately? Special attention should be given the marginal/average cost issue (e.g., hospital services), future costs, and the allocation of indirect costs.
3. Is a sensitivity analysis conducted on those costs that are uncertain?

A few studies have been selected for the reader to critically review. These are offered solely for the purpose of review and analysis; their selection is neither an endorsement nor a condemnation. These studies encompass:

1. evaluating costs in clinical trials;[11-13]
2. assessing the costs of treatment alternatives, using decision trees and outcome probabilities;[14,15] and
3. determining costs and benefits in societal economic evaluations.[16,17]

References

1. Wonnacott P, Wonnacott R. An introduction to microeconomics, 2nd ed. New York: McGraw-Hill, 1982.
2. Drummond MF, Stoddart GL, Torrance GW. Methods for the economic evaluation of health care programmes. Oxford: Oxford University Press, 1986. (Especially Ch. 3: Critical assessment of economic evaluation and Ch. 4: Cost analysis)
3. Guyatt G, Drummond M, Feeny D, et al. Guidelines for the clinical and economic evaluation of health care technologies. *Soc Sci Med* 1986;*22*:393-408.
4. Levin HM. Cost-effectiveness analysis in evaluation research. In: Guttentag M, Struening EL, eds. Handbook of evaluation research. Vol 2. Beverly Hills: Sage Publications, 1975:89-122.
5. Cleverly WO. Essentials of hospital finance. Germantown, MD: Aspen, 1978:81-95.
6. Neuhauser D, Lewicki AM. What do we gain from the sixth stool guaiac? *N Engl J Med* 1975;*293*:226.
7. Spiro HT. Finance for the nonfinancial manager. New York: John Wiley & Sons, 1977:98-109.
8. Berman HJ, Weeks LE. The financial management of hospitals, 3rd ed. Ann Arbor, MI: Health Administration Press, 1976:88-110.
9. Gagnon JP. Prescription department cost analysis. *Pharm Manage* 1979;*151*:235-40.
10. Roberts MJ. Work measurement. In: Brown TR, Smith MC, eds. Handbook of institutional pharmacy practice, 2nd ed. Baltimore: Williams & Wilkins, 1986:90-110.
11. Gill MA, Chenella FC, Heseltine PNR, et al. Cost analysis of antibiotics in the management of perforated or gangrenous appendicitis. *Am J Surg* 1986;*151*:200-4.
12. Thompson MS, Read JL, Hutchings C, Paterson M, Harris ED. The cost effectiveness of auranofin: results of a randomized clinical trial. *J Rheumatol* 1988;*15*:35-42.
13. Goodwin PJ, Feld R, Evans WK, Pater J. Cost-effectiveness of cancer chemotherapy: an

economic evaluation of a randomized trial in small-cell lung cancer. *J Clin Oncol* 1988;*6*:1537-47.

14. Stamm WE, McKevitt M, Counts GW, Wagner KF, Turck M, Holmes KK. Is antimicrobial prophylaxis of urinary tract infections cost effective? *Ann Intern Med* 1981;*94*:251-5.

15. Tsevat J, Durand-Zaleski I, Pauker SG. Cost-effectiveness of antibiotic prophylaxis for dental procedures in patients with artificial joints. *Am J Public Health* 1989;*79*:739-43.

16. Weinstein MC. Estrogen use in postmenopausal women—costs, risks, and benefits. *N Engl J Med* 1980;*303*:308-16.

17. Oster G, Epstein AM. Cost-effectiveness of antihyperlipemic therapy in the prevention of coronary heart disease: the case of cholestyramine. *JAMA* 1987;*258*:2381-7.

4

Health Status Indices and Quality of Life Assessment

Ronald W. Hansen

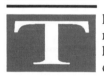he previous chapter discussed techniques to value items with market prices. Unfortunately, many of the events or services in health-related activities do not have a ready market. One cannot directly purchase recovery from a heart attack or freedom from pain. One may be able to place a value on the resources used to help a patient recovering from a heart attack or purchase a drug that will relieve pain. The question of interest often is not just to the value of resources devoted to healthcare, but to value the change in health status achieved by these interventions.

The problem of nonmarketed outcomes is not unique to the health sector. In fact, many publicly provided goods and services do not have a market price. Parks, police services, judicial systems, and many other services are provided with little or no cost to the user. Even when user fees are collected, they may bear little relation to the value of the services or the cost of providing the service. Rational decision-making or prudent stewardship of resources requires the development of methods to determine whether the services received justify the costs of providing them. The absence of an explicit market for these services complicates but does not eliminate the basic problem of trying to allocate scarce resources to their highest valued uses. Economists have developed a variety of methods to assign values to nonmarketed activities. Some methods involve surveys to measure the value respondents place on the service, but there are many problems related to potential respondent bias to opinion surveys. Other methods involve attempting to measure consumers' preferences or values as revealed in choices they make in related activities, or when faced with implicit costs of using a service. For example, a new park may be utilized by 25 of every 100 people who live within a 10-mile radius of the park, but by only 10 of every 100 people who live between 10 and 20 miles from the park, even though there is no comparable facility within the region. The decline in usage as the travel costs (both time and monetary) increase can be used to estimate the value that consumers place on the park services. In many instances, consumers reveal their value of nonmarketed services through their choices in related activities.

Using a variety of measures, economists have attempted to quantify health outcomes in terms of dollars. For many observers, the very attempt to quantify health outcomes in terms of monetary units is inappropriate, offensive, and perhaps immoral. Other observers accept the monetary measure in principle, but focus on methodological problems in the measures that have been employed. These problems are viewed as so severe as to make the estimates misleading for resource allocation. If one rejects quantifying health outcomes in monetary terms, but remains committed to trying to allocate resources efficiently, what options are available?

One solution is to resort to cost-effectiveness analysis, a technique described in Chapter 5. Basically, the technique allows one parameter, such as a particular health outcome, to remain in nonmonetary terms while measuring all other parameters in monetary terms. One then compares the dollar values expended (or received) to the changes in the other parameter. This technique can be a very valuable framework for analysis, particularly for finding the most efficient program to achieve a given objective or the maximum benefit to be received for a given expenditure. It often requires the decision maker to judge whether the level of benefit received is worth the cost, a feature that may be viewed as a virtue or vice, depending on one's view of the decision maker.

The cost-effectiveness framework loses some of its appeal if there are two or more nonmonetary parameters. With multiple parameters it is likely that for a given level of expenditure, no one program will dominate all parameters. The decision maker must weigh dollar costs against alternative sets of nonmonetary outcomes. As the number of these other parameters multiplies, the decision maker faces an increasingly complex problem. A solution to this dilemma is to assign relative weights to the nonmonetary parameters in order to collapse them to a single parameter, or at least to a small number of parameters. The assignment of relative weights often is a difficult and controversial task, especially since variations in the weighting system may radically change program decisions. It is essential that the basis for assignment of weights be well understood.

Several health status indices have been developed that potentially are useful in cost-benefit or cost-effectiveness studies. These indices provide a method to measure health states or treatment outcomes. The many dimensions of health are collapsed into a small number of parameters. In this chapter we provide an overview of health indices, discuss fundamental design issues, and describe some specific measures in greater detail. The chapter concludes with examples of the application of health indices in the evaluation of pharmaceuticals and pharmaceutical services.

Overview of Health Indices: Mortality and Morbidity

We employ the term "health index" as a generic term for a wide variety of measures related to health status, quality of life (QOL), or therapeutic outcomes. As their name implies, health indices are designed to measure a health event, but the specific measures differ greatly. The measures range from the simple to the complex, from individual to group characteristics, from point-in-time to lifetime, and from self-assessed to external evaluation. These differences reflect, in part, differences in their intended uses, including general descriptive devices, a tool for evaluating the effectiveness of treatment modalities, or an aid in selecting therapy for a particular patient.

The simplest and earliest indices of health status are measures of morbidity and mortality. Mortality indices are often easy to construct. The outcome measured, death, is a well-defined event, despite recent advances in life-support systems which have created new concepts of death for a small number of patients. Because deaths often are recorded, it is possible to construct mortality tables for many different groups, historical as well as contemporary.

Mortality data can be used to construct measures of the average lengths of lives, distribution of lengths of lives, or expected lifetimes for population groups. Another popular measure is the death rate per unit of population (e.g., deaths per million). Because mortality rates may be skewed by differences in age distributions, one may wish to construct an age-adjusted mortality index, a measure that may be more difficult than it first appears. For example, if one population has a high infant mortality rate but long life expectancy for those who survive their early years, and another has a low infant death rate but relatively higher rates among individuals in their middle-age years, methods used for constructing age-adjusted mortality rates may result in opposite rankings of the two populations.

Mortality statistics may use cause of death as a differentiating variable. This method requires determination of the cause of death and introduces conceptual problems as well as a greater likelihood of recording errors. There may be multiple events leading to death and it may be difficult to specify only one as the cause. Errors in diagnosis or record keeping may introduce further error into these measures. Random errors pose fewer problems than systematic errors generated by social or economic concerns. The social stigma that some associate with AIDS or suicide has resulted in some deaths due to these causes being given other classifications. Benefit programs for victims of particular diseases, such as black lung, may generate an increase in the recording of deaths due to these diseases.

But despite these problems, death rates by cause of death can be very useful for a variety of epidemiologic studies or as a descriptive device. For example, differences in incidence of death due to particular cancers or heart conditions across populations may be related to variations in diet or lifestyles and generate clues about the factors responsible for particular diseases.

Another mortality index frequently used in assessing alternative therapies is the survival rate through time. For example, in assessing two treatments for a particular type of cancer, one may produce an 80 percent survival rate after two years and the alternative therapy results in a two-year survival rate of only 70 percent. Viewed from this perspective, therapy that produces a higher survival rate could be judged superior to alternative therapies. Again, this simple assessment is confounded if the survival rate patterns are such that reversals occur. These hypothetical therapies may result in a five-year survival rate of 30 percent for the first therapy and 50 percent for the second. Straightforward survival rate analysis does not give a clear preference for either of the therapies. One solution is to calculate total life years following the two therapies. This calculation of total life years implicitly values each life year equally. Some evidence suggests that many individuals would prefer a two-year extension of life to a 50 percent probability of either immediate death or four years of survival.[1]

Morbidity indices are closely related to measures of death by cause. These indices typically measure the incidence of particular disease or disability and may be adjusted for age or other population characteristics. Like causation-specific mortality indices, they also are subject to misdiagnosis or difficulties related to multiple conditions. Unlike mortality indices, there often are problems of measuring the severity of the disease or disability. Pneumonia, influenza, and ulcers range from temporary discomforts to life-threatening illnesses. It may be possible to give a clinical measure of severity, but incorporating this into a morbidity index may be difficult. Other conditions are difficult even to clinically evaluate. For example, back pain has varying degrees of severity but it is not easy to measure the severity of the condition. However, to the extent that reliable morbidity indices can be constructed, they may be employed in much the same manner as causation-specific mortality indices.

Variation in the severity of conditions raises an evaluation problem not generally associated with mortality statistics. Even if only one disability is under consideration, one may face the problem of evaluating the relative importance of the disability's severity. For example, if we agree on a measure of the extent of vision loss, perhaps in percentage terms, is one 50 percent vision loss equal to two 25 percent losses? Or are two 50 percent losses equal to one total blindness?

Morbidity and mortality indices usually do not attempt to measure the value of alternative outcomes, but only the incidence or levels. They tend to be primarily descriptive in nature and do not attempt to assign relative importance to health states. As a descriptive device, these indices have very important analytical uses, but do not provide sufficient information for many health-policy questions.

Overview of Health Indices: Multiple Health States

In healthcare, one frequently encounters multidimensional decisions. A therapy that relieves pain may generate an increase in the risk of ulcers. An alternative therapy may not cause ulcers but may be somewhat less effective in relieving pain, and impairs vision in some patients. One may face the decision of expanding a coronary care unit or using the funds for prenatal care. The health outcomes are very different and may have impact on different people. One should be concerned that traditional measures, such as mortality indices, do not reflect QOL. Measures reflecting the multiplicity of health states and QOL are required to address issues involving complex health alternatives.

It would be difficult to point to a single beginning for work on multidimensional health status or QOL indices. Rosser traced the first health indicator to the Laws of Hammurabi, 1792 B.C., which spell out that the value of medical intervention depends on the actual outcome and socioeconomic class of the person who experiences the outcome. Rosser constructed a utility scale adjusted for socioeconomic groups based on these laws. The use of these indicators ended in 1750 B.C. and the next application of health indicators noted by Rosser occurred during the Victorian era. Florence Nightingale used a simple classification of "dead, relieved, or unrelieved" in her design for collecting hospital statistics. Rosser claims that "Nightingale was perhaps the first person to achieve changes, for example in hospital design, as a consequence of her health indicator."[2]

The modern era of health indicators is only about 20 years old. Rosser[3] credited Sullivan[4,5] for bringing rigor to the growing literature on the quality of healthcare and for proposing three health indices. The potential usefulness of improved health indices was recognized by several distinct researchers and multidisciplinary groups. These researchers have diverse interests, including concerns with describing the course of particular diseases to evaluating broad healthcare programs. This diversity in interest resulted in a multiplicity of health status indicators. We briefly describe the general types of indices in this section.

One perceived use was to better describe the ability or inability of individuals suffering from specific diseases to perform various functions. These functional indices have much in common with morbidity indices in that they are primarily descriptive, but provide much more detail about the extent of disability. The indices range from physical measures (e.g., movement of an arthritic joint) to the ability to perform activities of daily living (e.g., dressing or toileting).

Some individuals extended the functional indices to include social as well as physical factors. These studies recognized that the disease or disability may affect not only physical functioning, but also the ability to interact with one's environment. As the functional measures are expanded to include more mental health or social interaction variables, they take on more characteristics of the multidimensional health status indices.

As their name implies, multidimensional health status indices include many aspects of an individual's health status, such as outward signs of disease, symptoms expressed by the patient, and functions.[6] Many dimensions of health are included, but often little is done to collapse the descriptive material into a single-dimension scale.

As noted earlier, one of the concerns for evaluating healthcare programs is the necessity to compare, usually in some value sense, different types of medical conditions or therapeutic outcomes. This evaluation requires that the multidimensional measures be collapsed into a single or at least a few manageable dimensions. Conceptually, one needs to find a way to place relative weights on the dimensions, reflecting their contribution to the overall value system. For those dimensions that have resulted in a single parameter, that measure has been: (1) an index with no necessary linkage to other values; (2) an individual's utility, potentially comparable to utility derived from goods and services; or (3) a monetary measure, often derived from a willingness-to-pay model.

Fundamental Issues in Developing Health Indices

Many fundamental issues must be addressed in the construction of health indices. These issues relate to how health is to be defined and measured, the properties of the scale used, whose evaluation of the relative values of health states should be used, and the possibility of linking the health values to values for other goods or services. In this section, we discuss these conceptual and operational features followed by descriptions of the major indices in terms of their approaches to these features.

DEFINING HEALTH

Before attempting to measure health or changes in health, one must address the question of defining health. Is health merely the absence of overt illness or does it relate to such characteristics as strength, stamina, and alertness? Should perfect health refer to a standard few of us will ever achieve? Or should the base point be an average level of stamina, strength, etc., with no known signs of specific illness? Should health status refer only to one's physical characteristics or should one's mental state or ability to interact in a social context be included?

The concept of health may be affected by cultural factors. Ideal weight is, in part, culturally determined and even estimates based on the effect of weight on morbidity and mortality have been revised periodically. The ideal level of strength may be affected by the normal daily activities of the population. Not only is there no agreement as to what constitutes ideal health, there is some dispute about the other end of the spectrum. Many models use death as the ultimate lower bound. But some people believe that certain life states are worse than death. Kind et al.[7] and Torrance[8] have investigated incorporating states worse than death in health indices.

The World Health Organization has defined health as "a state of complete physical, mental, and social well-being, and not merely the absence of disease or infirmity."[9] Use of this definition would require a broad measure of well-being and not just a focus on the presence or absence of particular diseases. However, broad definitions such as this are too abstract to provide an operational focus for measuring health. As noted by one researcher, the difficulty in conceptualizing health is a major obstacle in developing and utilizing health status indicators.[6]

BREADTH OF MEASURE

The difficulty in precisely defining health relates to its multidimensional nature. It should not be surprising that in determining what should be incorporated into a measure of health, several dimensions have been suggested. An individual's sense of well-being, clinical evaluations, and ability to function are dimensions of health that appear in many of the health indices.

In discussing concepts of health in his review of health status indicators, Jette categorizes measures as operationalizing one or more of the following conceptual foci:[6]

1. Symptom/feeling states: phenomena experienced by an individual that are not directly observable by another person (e.g., pain, dizziness)
2. Signs: directly observable events that are evidence of illness (e.g., elevated blood pressure)
3. Performance: capacity or actual level of function

These conceptual foci are very broad and permit a great variety of measurement tools. Jette argues that in order to be useful as a generic health indicator, the measure should incorporate all three conceptual foci: symptom/feeling states, signs and performance.[6] Otherwise the measure describes something less than total health. Evaluation indicators can be more limited and focus on those dimensions affected by the program or disease.

WHOSE VALUES

Health indicators frequently are employed in assessment of programs with multidimensional medical outcomes. The indicators often compare these outcomes to one or a small number of parameters. Implicit or explicit values or weights are assigned to different health states. In measures of health states, whose values should be used? Should the patient, and/or the family, be the value source? For decisions involving only or primarily the patient, a strong case can be made for the patient's perspective. But rarely are the patient and immediate family the only parties affected by the healthcare decision. For major medical events, most care is financed through a third party, either a government program or private insurance. The financial burden of the care is shared by other members of the community. Particularly when government programs are involved, one can argue that the weights used in comparing medical outcomes should be those of the community. A third alternative is to rely on expert opinion. Just as patients often are willing to allow their physicians to select the best therapy for them, perhaps we should allow experts to make choices about the value of different health states. The determination of whose values should be used in establishing health measures will depend, in part, on the intended use of the measure.

Even if we were able to resolve the issue of whether private or community values should be used, we should consider the point in time at which these values should be assessed. When one is well, one can abstractly discuss the weights that should be assigned to different states of health. However, when one is afflicted by a particular illness, one's values may change. The decisions made at the bedside may differ from the ones made in the armchair. Even the larger community may be influenced by media attention to a particular patient or disease.

If agreement is reached that patient values should form the basis for evaluation, one still must face the question of whether the values should be those of a specific patient or an average of all patients. If the health index is being used to help determine the appropriate course of therapy for a specific patient, then the relative values that patient would place on the possible outcomes would be the appropriate basis of evaluation. The use of average values could result in selection of a therapy that would not be best suited for a particular patient.

In other situations, the same therapy will be used on all patients in the population, independent of their particular preferences, and these preferences will not affect the therapeutic results. In this situation, using average values for all patients generally will be appropriate, although for some types of scales averages are not meaningful.

In many cases, more than one therapy may be available for treatment of a particular disease or disability. The choice of specific therapy for a given patient often is affected by patient-specific characteristics, including his own preferences. This partial self-selection of therapies, based on patient preferences, poses a serious problem in evaluating therapeutic alternatives.

To the extent that average patient values are appropriate, one must construct different averages for the patients who self-select each therapy. One should not be startled to discover that a particular therapy may be the best for the patients who utilize it, but be less preferred for patients using alternative therapies. This may generate confidence in a system in which patient preferences can affect therapeutic choices. However, if one examines the literature, many assessments of alternative therapies use a single weighting scheme and ignore the possibility of alternative rankings of therapies based on individual preferences.

SCALING ISSUES

An issue that is both conceptual as well as operational is the selection of the type of scale to be used in measuring health. The scale or measuring system can be classified as nominal, ordinal, or cardinal. A nominal scale categorizes items by some characteristics, but generally does not attach any preference ordering. For example, we could categorize items by color, but the measure does not attach any relative value to green as opposed to red items. An external evaluator may use his own criteria for selecting among the groups, even though the scaling measure does not provide a relative ranking.

In contrast, an ordinal scale allows one to rank items, but does not require a measure of the degree of difference. For example, if preferences for particular items were being measured and we wanted to express the fact that item X is preferred to item Y, which is preferred to item Z, we could assign higher numbers to more preferred items, e.g., assigning the numbers 10, 9, and 8 to X, Y, and Z; or the numbers 15, 3, and 2. Either ranking expresses the preference ordering, but we are not able to make inferences about how much X is preferred to Y or Z.

For many evaluation purposes, we want a cardinal measure that not only gives us rankings, but is scaled to measure the amount of difference between alternatives. There are two types of cardinal measures: integer and ratio. Equal differences on an integer scale represent equal differences in the attribute being measured. For example, the attribute difference between items ranked 2 and 4 is the same as the difference between items ranked 8 and 10. But we cannot infer that the item ranked 4 has twice as much of the attribute as the one ranked 2. For example, the commonly used temperature scales are integer scales. The heat differential between 2 and 4 °C is the same as between 8 and 10 °C. But 4 °C is not twice as hot as 2 °C. In fact, using the Fahrenheit scale, the temperatures ranked 2 and 4 °C would be approximately 36 and 39 °F.

A ratio scale is a cardinal scale that measures the relative amount of the attribute. Thus, an item ranked 4 on the scale would contain twice the attribute level of an item ranked 2. Whereas the zero point on an integer scale need not have any special significance (e.g., 0 °F), a ratio scale must indicate the absence of the attribute being measured. A ratio scale is much more useful in analysis, but often is difficult to conceptualize and derive.

Is it possible to measure health on a ratio scale or are we limited to ordinal measures? It is tempting to ask individuals to rank health states along a scale and to then treat the scale as though it has integer or ratio properties when, in fact, the individual only was expressing an ordinal ranking. Consider a respondent facing two scales, the first from 0 to 1 and the second from 1 to 2; he places a particular health state in the midpoint of each scale and a second health state at 0.75 and 1.75 on the respective scales. If one were to interpret the scales as integer scales, the second health state would be equally different from the first and the top of both scales. In terms of a ratio scale, the second state is 50 percent greater than the first using the 0–1 scale and only 16⅔ percent greater using the 1–2 scale. Not only do the results depend on the scale used, but the respondent may only have been expressing the order of preference, with little thought to degree of preference.

Does it make sense to discuss health states in ratio terms? Can one state be considered twice the level of another, e.g., how healthy is an individual with mild hypertension compared to an individual recovering from a heart attack? Twice? Three times? Similar issues are faced in economics in trying to measure consumer satisfaction or utility. For most purposes, consumer choice theory only requires an ordinal measure of utility, but for some purposes, a ratio scale is desirable. A technique for constructing a ratio scale for utility has been employed in scaling health indices by using probability theory. Essentially, individuals faced the choice of receiving one outcome with certainty or accepting a gamble which, if won, would yield a preferred item, but if lost would result in no reward. The individuals then were offered various probabilities of winning the gamble and asked to select either the certain event or the gamble. The probability that made individuals indifferent between the two choices could be used to construct utility indices with integer properties. As we describe later, some researchers have used this basic technique to construct an integer-scaled health index.

Scaling issues are addressed by Brooks in a monograph. He provides an excellent summary of issues and a useful guide to the literature on this subject.[10]

═══ LINKAGE TO OTHER VALUES

If one has successfully constructed a health index the question remains, is it possible to link this index to other values? For cost-effectiveness analysis, it is not necessary to do this formally, although at some point the decision-maker must make judgments about the value of changes in the health states. If one were to translate the health indices into a form that could be utilized in cost-benefit analysis, then one would attempt to measure the value of changes in the health index in terms of dollars.

One method pursued particularly by economists is to try to measure the willingness of individuals to pay for changes in health status. Some of these attempts are pursued via a questionnaire formation in which individuals are asked how much they are willing to pay for disease avoidance or treatments. These attempts are subject to many sources of bias. One principal source is the suspicion by respondents that their answer may affect how much they have to pay for treatments that change their health status. Those who link their answer to their required payment will be tempted to report a very low value for improvements in health status. If the same individuals were requested to assess the cost of incurring a decline in health status and their response was believed to affect their compensation for incurring this loss, the value placed on changed health status may be considerably higher. One may reduce this respondent bias by approaching the issue from both directions.

Another form of respondent bias is the social desirability bias. Individuals may consider it socially unacceptable to place a finite value on life, or at least they may consider it unacceptable to place anything but a very high value on life.

Rather than relying on what individuals say about the value of health status, economists have attempted to measure the value individuals appear to place on health by the actions and choices they make.[11,12] Many choices that individuals make about life styles, jobs, and the purchase of goods with varying safety characteristics, involve trading safety for other attributes, including dollars or income. Using these actual choices as a basis, economists have attempted to derive implicit values for health and safety.

For example, if an additional expenditure of $500 for a safety device on a machine would allow one to reduce the probability of a fatal accident involving the use of the machine by 1 in a 1000 over the life of the machine, the implicit cost of avoiding a fatal accident is $500 000 per accident. If the device does not affect the operation of the machine other than to reduce the accident rate, then individuals who voluntarily choose not to purchase the safety device are implicitly placing a value of less than $500 000 for avoidance of a fatal accident. Alternatively, individuals who purchase the device place an implicit value of at least $500 000 on the avoidance of a fatal accident.

This calculation of value per fatal accident avoided requires several assumptions. First is linearity in the valuation of risk, for example, 100 reductions in risk by 1 in 100 is as valuable as eliminating one occurrence of the event. Another major assumption is that individuals understand the nature of the risk and can make unbiased calculations about the probability of adverse events. Some individuals charge that risks are poorly understood, in part because the average individual is not supplied with the actuarial data or conclusions necessary to assign risk to particular products or activities. The other basis for attack is the assertion supported by some studies that individuals have difficulty processing information about low-probability high-cost events, or that individuals are myopic when dealing with the probability of their own death. Work by Kahneman and Tversky has shown that, even when individuals try to be logical, they may give radically different answers depending on how the question is posed.[13]

These criticisms cannot be dismissed lightly and one should be cautious in placing great weight on a study involving only a single decision point or conducted in contexts in which risks are difficult to assess. However, by examining a variety of situations in which individuals make choices involving risk of death or injury, one may be able to draw reasonable estimates about the value individuals in practice place on life and limb.

===== COST UTILITY

Another technique to link health indices to other values is to attempt to measure the contribution of health status to an individual's utility. Utility is a concept used by economists to measure satisfaction or well-being and forms the basis for many models of consumer choice. Consumers derive varying amounts of utility or satisfaction from goods and services and their choice of goods or services depends on the amount of utility received compared with the expenditure required to obtain the good. Consumers will purchase the goods that give them the greatest utility per dollar spent. Cost-utility analysis attempts to measure the utility derived from changes in health status and to calculate the cost per unit of utility. Alternative programs can be compared on this basis and health programs can be compared with other areas of consumer purchases.

The major difficulty in constructing and utilizing cost-utility indices is that there is no agreement on a scale for measuring utility. For most of the economic models of consumer choice, it is necessary only to rank order choices, a criterion that can be satisfied by a variety of utility scales. The problems of constructing a utility scale are similar to those discussed in the next section regarding scales used in health indices.

Specific Design Issues

Once one has determined the conceptual basis for the construction of a health index, there are several issues related to the specific design of the index. The principal criteria are the validity, reliability, and ease of administering the index. These issues frequently are encountered in survey research.

A variety of validity measures are employed, the principal ones being content validity, construct validity, and discriminant validity.[14-16] Content validity refers to whether the instrument, in fact, measures what it claims to. Does it address the proper domains and are appropriate weights given to the items in the index? Construct (or convergent) validity is an evaluation of the relationship between the results of the measure in question and other related measures. To test construct validity one must have an idea about how the different measures ought to be related. Discriminant validity usually refers to the ability to discriminate between different events.

Kaplan et al. discussed the above concepts of validity and applied them to their index of well-being. In addition they consider criterion validity, the extent that the index corresponds to an observation that accurately measures the phenomenon of interest. The criterion must be a superior measure of the phenomena in question. They argue that no well-defined criteria exists for health and their criterion validity cannot be assessed.[14]

One should be careful to note that validity should be assessed within the context of the particular intended use. A measure that has demonstrated validity in one context may not be equally valid in another. Brooks warns that statements made about validity of particular measures should be examined critically because a certain degree of salesmanship is involved.[15]

Reliability, stability, and internal consistency are interrelated concepts, and there are a variety of methods to test for these properties. Does repeated administration to the same population yield similar results? Do the results differ when used by different raters? Are the responses internally consistent?

Indices differ considerably in the difficulty of administration. Indices requiring clinical measurements and in-depth personal interview generally are the most difficult and costly to administer. These indices usually require extensive training for those conducting the interview as well as an extended time commitment from both the interviewer and respondent. At the other extreme are self-administered questionnaires with a small number of easily understood questions.

Proper survey research techniques and questionnaire design are important skills for health status and QOL assessment. Clinical practitioners are encouraged to collaborate with health services researchers and pharmacy administration colleagues who can assist in these aspects of pharmacoeconomic methods.

Alternative Methods of Valuing Health Status or Changes in Health Status

As noted earlier, many health indices have been constructed and some have undergone a series of revisions. We will not attempt to describe or even list all of the indices. Among the more extensive reviews of indices are those of Jette[6] and Brooks.[15] We will concentrate our attention on a few of the better-known indices in each class.

FUNCTIONAL INDICES

Functional indices usually are applied in the context of specific disabilities such as arthritis, stroke, and the general aging process. One of the frequently cited class or functional indices is the activities of daily living (ADL).[17] The arthritis impact measurement scale is a specific application of ADL measures.[18] These indices measure the patient's ability to perform basic functions such as bathing, dressing, feeding, and toileting. Instrumental ADLs are broader in nature and include measures of other common activities such as telephone use and money management. Some functional indices have expanded to include social aspects of daily functions and resemble more comprehensive health status measures.

The particular items included in functional indices usually are measurable using an ordinal scale, but most cannot be easily placed in a cardinal scale. Even though the individual items can be ranked ordinally, most functional scales are not amenable to an overall ordinal ranking because there is no weighting of the relative importance of particular functions. For some measures, an overall score is presented by adding the individual rankings. One should be cautious in using such an overall score without investigating the basis for the weights assigned to each component.

Many components of functional indices can be evaluated by the test administrator while observing the subject performing tasks or measured by more traditional self-reported means. The time required for administering the test instrument obviously depends on the method selected.

HEALTH PROFILES

There are several indices that provide a profile of the respondent's health and include functional as well as social and emotional variables. Among these are the sickness impact profile (SIP)[19] and the general health rating index (GHRI) used in the Rand Insurance study.[20]

The health profiles are intended to provide a description of the patient's health in a variety of dimensions. Some provide a score for each section of the profile and others provide an overall score. Caution is advised in using the overall scores. They have been used to measure the impact of medical interventions or insurance programs on these different aspects of patient health.

The health profiles generally rely on self-reporting through personal interview or self-administered instruments, although the functional components could be obtained by direct observation. The ease of administration depends, in part, on the number of items included. In a comparison of the SIP, the GHRI and the quality of well-being scale (QWB) (discussed in the next section), Read et al. assessed the validity and ease of administration for these instruments. All three instruments scored well on the validity tests. The GHRI was the easiest to administer primarily because it is self-administered. The interviewer-administered version of the SIP required more extensive interviewer training (one week) and was somewhat longer and more difficult to administer. The QWB is also administered by the interviewer and requires the longest training time for interviewers (one to two weeks) due to the branching structure of its questions.[16]

AGGREGATED MULTIATTRIBUTE INDICES

Some indices are designed to produce a single score that can be particularly useful in cost-effectiveness evaluations. The QWB and the utility-based scales developed by Kind et al.[7] and Torrance[21] are examples of these indices.

The QWB index is divided into four sections: symptom-problem complex, mobility, physical function, and social function. The responses for each section result in a score that when aggregated gives an overall well-being score. The possible scores range from 0 (death) to 1 (perfect health). Unlike the health profiles discussed above, this aggregate score is the outcome intended for further use.

In its extended use, the QWB scale is treated as having integer and ratio properties. For example, this scale is used to construct quality-adjusted life years resulting from alternative programs or treatments. Basically, the QWB score is multiplied by the number of years an individual survives in that state to produce a well-years score. For some treatment programs, the person may pass through several different health states and the time spent in each state is adjusted by the QWB score. In this use, a treatment that has a four-year survival rate with a QWB score of 0.3 is equivalent to a treatment with a two-year survival rate and a QWB score of 0.6.

The utility-based indices also are intended to produce a score with integer properties. Culyer[22] and Read et al.[16] have investigated the construction of utility indices using both the standard gamble approach and a time-trade-off approach. As described earlier, this approach involves confronting the respondent with the choice of one event with certainty or the probability of obtaining one of two alternative events. If we use a scale in which death and perfect health are the two anchors, then we can rate health states using the probability of death versus perfect health at which they are indifferent between this gamble and the certainty of the specified health state (Figure 1). The lower the probability of death required to obtain indifference, the higher the value of the health state. Torrance has extended the approach to consider states worse than death or to model temporary health states.[8,21] Figures 2 and 3 illustrate the standard gamble alternatives for these situations.[23]

A similar scaling technique is provided by the time-trade-off model developed by Torrance.[23] Rather than the probability variable, these models look at trade-offs between the length of time spent in particular health states. An individual is offered two alternatives, t years of life with a chronic condition followed by death or health for a period x followed by death (Figure 4).[23]

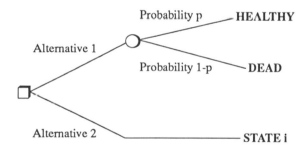

Figure 1. Standard gamble for a chronic health state preferred to death.[23]

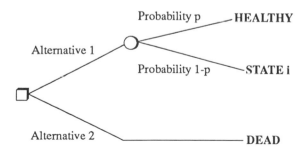

Figure 2. Standard gamble for a chronic health state considered worse than death.[23]

The value of x for which the respondent is indifferent is used to construct a preference value for that state:

$$h = \left(\frac{x}{t}\right)$$ **Eq. 1**

This formulation is used where the chronic health state is preferable to death. Torrance has modified this basic technique to study states worse than death or temporary states.[8,21]

Health Indices and Studies of Pharmaceuticals

Much of the literature on health indices has focused on the development and testing of the indices. Although the traditional morbidity and mortality indices have been used extensively in cost-benefit and cost-effectiveness analyses, the more recent indices have not yet found wide use in cost analyses. Utilization of the concept of quality-adjusted life years is growing in cost studies involving therapies for chronic conditions. Although pharmaceuticals are often part of therapy

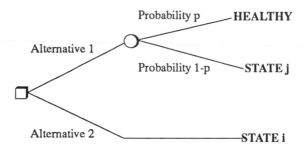

Figure 3. Standard gamble for a temporary health state.[23]

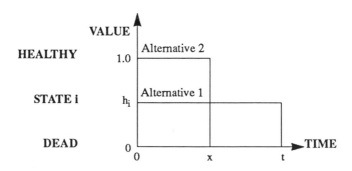

Figure 4. Time trade-off for a chronic health state preferred to death.[23]

regimens studied, very few studies employing these indices for specific pharmaceutical products or services are available. One might expect more such literature to be published. We discuss studies that have been performed in three therapeutic areas.

RHEUMATIC DISEASES

One index used to evaluate drug therapies is the arthritis impact measurement scale (AIMS). As described by Meenan, "Work on the Arthritis Impact Measurement Scales was begun in 1978 in an attempt to develop a more arthritis-specific health status measure, with the express intention of producing a useful tool for the evaluation of therapeutic and programmatic interventions in the rheumatic disease." He argues that in addition to evidence of traditional clinical and laboratory evidence of disease activity, "the AIMS instrument, or a similar functional approach, should become a standard component of drug evaluations in the rheumatic diseases." Note that the use he is proposing is primarily directed at the effectiveness studies to obtain drug approval rather than at cost-based studies.[18] However, establishing the AIMS instrument in this manner would lead to the possibility of employing it in cost-based studies.

During their clinical trials of auranofin, an oral gold agent for rheumatoid arthritis, Smith Kline & French investigated the effect of the drug on QOL. It was recognized that the drug was likely to increase drug and office visit costs and possibly total treatment cost over the short run. They were interested in determining whether the product generated any measurable effect on the QOL.[24]

As reported by Paterson, the study involved a comparison of auranofin with a control therapy likely to be employed.[24] The two QOL measures used were the Fries et al. health assessment questionnaire[25] and the Kaplan and Bush quality of well-being questionnaire.[26] An outside organization, Rhode Island Health Services Research, supervised the study. The study involved a comparison of baseline values and values six months later. In results presented at the American Rheumatism Association Annual Scientific Meeting in June 1985, auranofin produced greater improvement in all four of the composite health-status measures and with statistically significant changes in three of the four. The final results were presented in terms of dollars per quality-adjusted life year.[24]

CARDIOVASCULAR THERAPIES

Wenger et al. also argue for the inclusion of health index data in the assessment of therapies in clinical trials. They state, "The effect of cardiovascular interventions on these [quality-of-life] variables has not been examined in most clinical trials. Although patients and physicians often require information about the impact of therapy on quality-of-life to make a rational selection of treatment alternatives."[27]

In their study of hypertension, Weinstein and Stason consider the effects of strokes and myocardial infarction on the QOL as well as the length of life. They employed a methodology estimating the number of years individuals spend in various disability states following these events. QOL weights then are applied to the time in these disability states to measure QOL years lost due to stroke or myocardial infarctions. In their cost-effectiveness analysis of treatment protocols, including drug therapy, they are able to express their results in terms of cost per quality-adjusted life year. Their assessments include drug regimens, effects of medication noncompliance, and hypertension detection programs.[28-30]

Croog et al. studied the effects of three antihypertensive pharmaceuticals on QOL. Assessment was based on five groups of measures: (1) sense of well-being and satisfaction with life, (2) physical state, (3) emotional state, (4) intellectual functioning, and (5) ability to perform in social roles and the degree of satisfaction derived from those roles. To construct these measures, all or part of ten different indices were used. Their results are presented for specific measures as well as for aggregates. Baseline values were collected and compared with the values for these measures after 24 months. For many of the health indices, no significant differences were found among the three drugs. In other measurements, one drug dominated the other two.[31]

The authors did note the parallel between their recorded changes in general well-being index and differences found in studies of other conditions. Other than to assert that the changes in that index were clinically significant, no attempt was made to impute a value to any of the differences noted.[31]

ANTIHISTAMINES

In his Ph.D. dissertation, Reardon examined the use of contingent valuation and utility models for the assessment of the value of pharmaceuticals in treating allergic rhinitis. The principal contribution of the thesis was the testing of a contingent valuation methodology. He utilized a mail questionnaire in which respondents were asked a series of questions about their willingness to pay for relief of symptoms of allergic rhinitis and avoidance of medication adverse effects. This questionnaire included complete avoidance of effects as well as alternative combinations of relief and adverse effects resulting from the use of products with hypothesized characteristics. Respondents also were asked to express their degree of like or dislike for the hypothesized products. From this evidence, Reardon was able to derive values for product attributes and construct contingent valuation models. He concluded that "there is a positive relationship between measures of contingent valuation predicted by utility models and actual contingent valuation for the set of hold-out product profiles." The use of a mail questionnaire rather than direct interview reduced the administrative cost of the study.[32] It is expected that extensions of this work will result in applications of contingent valuation methodology to other areas of pharmaceutical services or products.

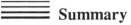
Summary

Given the complex nature of many questions in the healthcare arena, it is necessary to develop methods to evaluate the multiplicity of potential outcomes. The situation is further complicated by the difficulty in measuring some important outcomes, such as the improvement in an individual's sense of well-being. Many of the health-status indicators surveyed in this chapter may prove useful in addressing some of these questions. There is a need for the development and validation of these instruments targeted at specific disease states and specific drug classes. These focused questionnaires should have many advantages, including possibly shorter length and improved sensitivity to therapy response, which can make them more practical in their application to pharmacoeconomic studies.

One should take careful note that the indices have been designed for a variety of purposes and one should carefully select the measures best suited for the particular problem being addressed. Some are designed to describe health parameters but make no attempt to address relative values to changes in health states. Others are intended as measures of relative values that can be incorporated in cost-benefit and cost-effectiveness evaluations.

Measures such as the QWB instrument and its extension to the construction of QOL years measures provide a convenient but controversial tool for analysis. The weights implicit in the QWB index may not be appropriate either for the study population or as reflective of the values of the decision-maker. Some critics also find it repugnant to adjust life years by a quality index for assessment purposes. Others find it irresponsible not to make the adjustment. Appeal to health indices may mask but does not eliminate many of these fundamental issues in evaluation. Although it is unlikely that these issues will ever be resolved to everyone's satisfaction, health indices offer a reasonable approach that will become increasingly important.

References

1. McNeil BJ, Weichselbaum R, Pauker SG. Fallacy of the five-year survival in lung cancer. *N Engl J Med* 1978;*299*:1397-401.
2. Rosser RM. Issues of measurement in the design of health indicators: a review. In: Culyer AJ, ed. Health indicators. Oxford: Martin Robertson, 1983: 34-81.
3. Rosser RM. A history of the development of health indicators. In: Smith GT, ed. Measuring the social benefits of medicine. London: Office of Health Economics, 1983: 50-62.
4. Sullivan DF. Conceptual problems in developing an index of health. Washington, DC: U.S. Department of Health, Education and Welfare. Publication no. (HRA) 74-1017, series 2, no. 5, 1966.
5. Sullivan DF. A single index of mortality and morbidity. HMSHA Health Reports, 1971: 347-55.
6. Jette AM. Health status indicators: their utility in chronic disease evaluation research. *J Chronic Dis* 1980;*33*:567-79.

7. Kind P, Rosser R, Williams A. Valuation of quality of life: some psychometric evidence. In: Jones-Lee MW, ed. The value of life and safety. Amsterdam: North-Holland, 1982.

8. Torrance GW. Health states worse than death. In: van Elmeren W, Engelbrecht R, Flagle CD, eds. Third international conference on system science in health care. Berlin: Springer-Verlag, 1984:1085-9.

9. The first ten years of the World Health Organization. Geneva: World Health Organization, 1985.

10. Brooks RG. Scaling in health status measurement: an outline guide and commentary. Lund, Sweden: The Swedish Institute for Health Economics, 1988.

11. Thaler R, Rosen S. The value of saving a life: evidence from the labor market. *Household Prod Consum* 1975;*40*:265-302.

12. Viscusi WK. Labor market valuations of life and limb: empirical evidence and policy implication. *Public Policy* 1978;*26*:259-386.

13. Kahneman D, Tversky A. Choices, values, and frames. *Am Psychol* 1984;*39*:341-50.

14. Kaplan RM, Bush JW, Berry C. Health status: types of validity and the index of well-being. *Health Serv Res* 1976;*11*:478-507.

15. Brooks RG. The development and construction of health status measures: an overview of the literature. Lund, Sweden: The Swedish Institute for Health Economics, 1986.

16. Read JL, Quinn RJ, Hoefer MA. Measuring overall health: an evaluation of three important approaches. *J Chronic Dis* 1987;*40*(suppl):7S-21S.

17. Katz S. Assessing self-maintenance: activities of daily living, mobility and instrumental activities of daily living. *J Am Geriatr Soc* 1983;*31*:721-7.

18. Meenan RF. Assessing therapeutic effectiveness in the rheumatic diseases: the case for functional and health status measures. In: Symposia Medica Hoechst 16. Stuttgart: FK Schattauer, 1981: 353-64.

19. Bergner M, Kaplan RM, Ware JE Jr. Evaluating health measures (commentary). *J Chronic Dis* 1987;*40*(suppl):23S-6S.

20. Ware JE. Methodological considerations in the selection of health status assessment procedures. In: Wenger NK, Mattson ME, Furberg CD, et al., eds. Assessment of quality of life in clinical trials of cardiovascular therapies. New York: Le Jacq Publishing, 1984: 84-117.

21. Torrance GW. Multiattribute utility theory as a method of measuring social preferences for health states in long-term care. In: Kane RL, Kane RA, eds. Values and long-term care. Lexington, KY: Lexington Books, 1982:127-56.

22. Culyer AJ, ed. Health indicators. Oxford: Martin Robertson, 1983.

23. Torrance GW. Measurement of health state utilities for economic appraisal: a review. *J Health Econ* 1986;*5*:1-30.

24. Paterson ML. Measuring the socio-economic benefits of health care. In: Ekonomisk utvardering av mya lakemedel. Stockholm: RUFI, 1987.

25. Fries JF, Wasner C, Brown J, Feigenbaum P. A controlled trial of antihypertensive therapy in systemic sclerosis (sceleroderma). *Ann Rheum Dis* 1984;*43*:407-10.

26. Kaplan RM, Bush JW. Health-related quality of life measurement for evaluation research and policy analysis. *Health Psychol* 1982;*1*:61-80.

27. Wenger NK, Mattson ME, Furberg CD, Elinson J. Assessment of quality of life in clinical trials of cardiovascular therapies. In: Wenger NK, Mattson ME, Furberg CD, et al., eds. Assessment of quality of life in clinical trials of cardiovascular therapies. New York: LeJacq Publishing, 1984:1-22.

28. Weinstein MC, Stason WB. Allocation of resources to manage hypertension. *N Engl J Med* 1977;*296*:732-9.

29. Weinstein MC, Stason WB. Foundations of cost-effectiveness analysis for health and medical practices. *N Engl J Med* 1977;*296*:716-21.

30. Weinstein MC, Stason WB. Hypertension: a policy perspective. Cambridge, MA: Harvard University Press, 1976.

31. Croog SH, Levine S, Testa MA, et al. The effects of antihypertensive therapy on the quality of life. *N Engl J Med* 1986;*314*:1657-64.

32. Reardon G. Contingent valuation and utility models for economic evaluation of pharmaceuticals: a study of antihistamines (dissertation). Columbus: Ohio State University, 1987.

5

Cost-Effectiveness
Analysis

Elizabeth A. Chrischilles

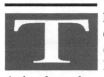he major objectives of this chapter are to: (1) define the concept and basic framework of cost-effectiveness analysis (CEA), (2) enumerate the steps involved in a proper CEA, and (3) illustrate these with examples from the drug therapy literature. At its close, the reader hopefully will have developed an appreciation for what CEA is, what it is not, and what it can be in the future. Since much of the terminology and concepts involved in CEA have been developed in previous chapters (e.g., direct/indirect costs, sensitivity analysis, discounting), these concepts will not be covered in depth. However, the reader can expect to find much discussion of the nuances of these same terms and concepts as they apply to CEA of drug therapy.

CEA Defined

Like cost-benefit analysis (CBA), CEA is an approach used for identifying, measuring, and comparing all the significant pros and cons of alternative health-care practices (interventions). With respect to drug therapy, these alternative interventions may be two or more different drugs or classes of drugs; or the goal may be to compare drug treatment with one or more types of nondrug treatment for a particular condition.

Unlike CBA, which values all effects of an intervention in dollar terms, CEA measures some effects in nonmonetary terms. The predominant approach used in CBA to value personal health benefits is the human capital approach. CEA, on the other hand, makes no attempt to do this. For this reason, some feel that CEA is less comprehensive than CBA, since it excludes the valuation of life.

However, the human capital approach of CBA also does not incorporate the value of life. In fact, CBA is not inherently more comprehensive than CEA since, even though it includes the market value of life, CBA excludes the nonmarket value of life. CEA, on the other hand, includes it, implicitly but quantitatively in nonmonetary measures such as life years saved, disability days avoided, quality-adjusted life years gained, and episodes of nephrotoxicity avoided. It is because of this nonmonetary measurement of health outcome that CEA cannot be used to compare interventions with different health outcomes. For example, if two drugs each have associated costs of $2000, but one prevents 100 days of disability and the other saves one life, CEA cannot be used to compare the two drugs because it does not provide a single metric along which to measure these very different outcomes.

Beyond these general statements, the definition of CEA becomes difficult due to its dynamic nature. Many analytical developments have occurred during recent years, resulting in several variations of the basic CEA framework. The appropriateness of each variation depends upon the drug therapy question that the analyst faces.

THE BASIC FRAMEWORK AND VARIATIONS ON THE THEME

The basic framework of CEA involves the comparison of the net resource effects (costs) of an intervention with some nonmonetary measure(s) of its net effect on health outcome (effectiveness). This frequently is expressed as the ratio of the two and is called a cost-effectiveness ratio. The resulting ratio takes the form of dollars per unit of effectiveness (e.g., dollars per life year saved).

Costs. In CEA, the costs of an intervention are better termed its net costs, which are a measure of the net effects of an intervention on resource use. As such, they consist not only of economic costs (resource use), but also economic benefits (resource savings). In other words, the resource effects of an intervention include production costs, induced resource losses, and induced resource savings. Production costs are the resources used to actually provide the intervention. Induced resource losses are the resources consumed in tests and treatments undertaken as a consequence of the initial intervention (e.g., due to adverse effects of the intervention). Induced resource savings are resource expenditures averted as a consequence of the initial intervention (e.g., from prevention of subsequent morbidity that would have required evaluation and treatment). Net costs of an intervention therefore are calculated as production costs plus induced resource losses minus induced resource savings. Induced resource savings are actually economic benefits that enter the net cost calculation as negative costs.

Production costs, induced resource losses, and induced resource savings include both direct and indirect costs and savings. Indirect costs and indirect savings have not typically been included in net cost calculations in the healthcare literature. Indirect costs include lost patient and family earnings due to time missed from work or reduced productivity while at work because of the intervention (for example, as a result of adverse drug effects or travel time to receive the intervention). Indirect savings are savings on indirect costs of illness (time and productivity losses associated with illness) due to the prevention or alleviation of disease by the intervention. The rationale for omission of indirect costs and savings from drug therapy CEAs has been that it is more consistent to include only the components of dollar costs that add to or subtract from the resources available for healthcare since these net costs are being compared with net health effectiveness.[1] However, these time and productivity losses and gains may have substantial financial consequences for individuals and society. It certainly would be possible to estimate all resource savings and costs, including the value of time and productivity losses and gains. In such a case, the nonmonetary effectiveness measure could be judged against a more comprehensive assessment of economic impacts.

One of the most controversial aspects of CEA is the issue of whether to include healthcare costs occurring in the added years of life. Some feel that these costs, which include the costs of treating diseases that would not have occurred if the patient had not lived longer as a result of the original intervention, should be incorporated.[1,2] Others feel that these should not be included, since this overestimates the costs associated with life-saving interventions.[3,4] Furthermore, it seems inconsistent to include consumption of healthcare resources in added years without including productivity and other types of consumption that also come with prolonged life.[3,4]

Health Effectiveness. The simplest version of health effectiveness is a single health effectiveness measure. Although health status is multidimensional, we often are concerned with a single health measure and the most efficient means of reaching it. For example, which of two drugs will produce the greatest number of cures per dollar spent? Here, the number of cures can serve as the single measure of health effectiveness. Similarly, a single measure for mortality could be the number of lives saved (or lost) by each intervention. Alternatively, the number of years of life or life expectancy that are added by a particular intervention can be calculated. A single health effectiveness measure can incorporate both the beneficial health effects (drug efficacy) and the negative health effects (drug toxicity) of the intervention. For example, in a study of the cost-effectiveness of antimicrobial choices for nosocomial pneumonia, Weinstein et al. combined each regimen's expected effects on mortality from infection with its expected effects on mortality from drug toxicity. These were combined to form the total expected loss in life expectancy for each regimen. The regimen with the lowest expected loss in life expectancy thus exhibited the highest net effectiveness.[5]

Another approach to measuring the health effectiveness of interventions is through the use of multiple health effectiveness measures. For example, rather than combine the beneficial and negative health effects of an intervention in a single nonmonetary unit of measure, each effect can be presented separately, often using different units of measure. For example, in a CEA of topical versus systemic agent treatment for papulopustular acne, Stern et al. expressed the trade-offs between costs and nonmonetary effects of the two regimens by displaying their results in table format. The systemic agent strategy had greater benefit (fewer weeks of morbidity from acne) and lower dollar cost; however, it had a nearly doubled risk of adverse effects from treatment.[6] An analogous situation occurs when an outcome has more than one relevant beneficial effect and it is difficult to combine these effects in a single measurement unit. For example, a medication may offer decreased morbidity but an increased mortality rate over surgical intervention. In such a situation, a proper analysis should reflect this trade- off between quality and length of life. An approach taken by some researchers is to separately present the effects of the interventions on longevity and quality of life (QOL). The principal difficulty with the use of multiple measures lies in the interpretation of results. If a particular intervention is more cost-effective according to each of two effectiveness measures, there is no difficulty in interpretation. The problem arises when an intervention is more cost-effective than the alternative(s) according to one effectiveness measure and less cost-effective according to the other. This was the case in the CEA of acne treatment described above. Since there is no common unit of measure, the decision becomes subjective and one must ask if it is more important to avoid morbidity from acne or adverse effects.

Other investigators have made use of combined health effectiveness measures to provide a common unit of measurement in situations involving trade-offs, such as between longevity and QOL. These combined measures explicitly incorporate the kind of value judgment just discussed. Probably the most used of such combined measures is the quality-adjusted life-year (QALY), where "the number of QALYs is the number of years at full health that would be valued equivalently to the numbers of years of life as experienced."[7] Since some years are typically at less than full health, due to morbidity from disease, the number of QALYs is smaller than the number of years experienced. For example, a year of full health would equal 1.0 QALY, whereas two years valued at 0.4 each, would count together as 0.8 QALY. The method by which value is assigned to a year at a given health status level involves utility assessment, which is discussed in Chapter 6. Weinstein and Fineberg have described these methods as they pertain to CEA. Briefly, the two approaches used to obtain these utility assessments are the time-trade-off method and the lottery method. Both measures involve eliciting from physician, patients, or others, subjective assessments of the desirability of health states. In the time-trade-off method, the following question is asked: If disability, lost earnings, limitation of activity, pain, and suffering are taken into account, what is the smallest fraction, P, of a year of life at full health that you would accept in exchange for a year of life at health status, S?[7]

The answer, P, becomes the value for a year of life as experienced (i.e., in the particular health status level). If P is close to 1, the health status is near full health. A value of P close to 0 implies that the particular health state is nearly as bad as death.[7]

As is obvious by the nature of the question that must be answered to assign these values, the QALY scale is subjective and suffers all the shortcomings of utility assessment. The predictions made from studies asking these types of questions of patients have been found to vary substantially from actual patient decisions. For this reason, many advocate more objective assessments of QOL, obtained in the context of controlled trials.[8,9] In addition to greater objectivity, an advantage of collecting empirical QOL data is that multiple measures that encompass the several domains of QOL can be used. If such empirical data are used, however, there is no rational way of converting that data into the values used in the QALY method; thus, a combined measure is no longer possible.

Another approach to providing a combined health effectiveness measure in the situation of multiple health outcomes is to use utility analysis to assign utility values for each possible outcome. The expected utility associated with each intervention then becomes the combined measure of health effectiveness. Results then are presented as dollar costs per utility for each intervention. The same objections have been raised for this approach as for the QALY method, since both rely on subjective and variable utility assessments. An example of this approach is a study by Nettlemen et al., in which the cost-effectiveness of using a cell culture to test for chlamydial infections was compared with empiric treatment in high- and low-risk patients. The possible outcomes are: cure with and without tetracycline adverse effects; no cure without complications, with and without tetracycline adverse effects; and no cure with complications, with and without tetracycline adverse effects. Complications were defined as pelvic inflammatory disease (women), ectopic pregnancy (women), infertility (women), and epididymitis (men). Adverse effects of tetracycline were nausea and vomiting and yeast infections (women). Utility values were assigned for each possible outcome and a decision-tree format was used to determine the expected utility for each intervention. The cost per utility was lowest for empiric treatment in both men and women, regardless of risk group, at a cost per utility of $15.64. The next most cost-effective protocol would be empiric treatment for patients at high-risk and culture-based treatment for women at low-risk, at a cost per utility of $31.71. The study did not quantitatively consider the negative social and psychological effects of a diagnosis (and, therefore, treatment) of a sexually transmitted disease. However, the authors observed that, although empiric treatment of all patients was associated with the lowest cost per utility, it might not be the most desirable approach given these social and psychological effects.[10]

MISUSE OF THE TERM

Cost-consciousness in healthcare has resulted in widespread use of the term cost-effective. Unfortunately, this has not been accompanied by a clear understanding of the term. Doubilet et al. have summarized the misuse of the term in the medical literature. Studies equating cost-effectiveness with cost savings and those declaring an intervention to be cost-effective based only on effectiveness data are equally erroneous. Either interpretation considers only half of the term.[11]

▤ RECOMMENDED USE OF THE TERM

Cost-effectiveness should be used to imply value for money. Table 1 illustrates very generally some possible combinations of cost and effectiveness that might be discovered with a CEA of drug A versus drug B. If the costs associated with drug A are lower than drug B and drug A is also more effective (cell X_3), drug A is clearly more cost-effective than drug B. Cell X_2 also has an obvious interpretation: drug B is more cost-effective than drug A in this case. Cells X_1 and X_4 are more difficult to interpret. In cell X_1, drug A is both more effective and more costly than drug B; in cell X_4, it is both less effective and less costly than drug B. In either case, one must consider whether having the additional effectiveness is worth the additional costs (or whether having the decreased cost is worth the decreased effectiveness). For example, in a study of the cost-effectiveness of antimicrobial choices for nosocomial pneumonia, Weinstein et al. estimated that ceftizoxime had a lower expected cost per patient, but would result in the loss of an additional 0.44 years of life expectancy compared with the regimen of mezlocillin plus gentamicin. They estimated that the latter regimen would cost an additional $1026 per year of life expectancy gained. These types of trade-offs between effectiveness and costs of care are a reality that must be faced. In the above case, the authors considered the increased effectiveness of the combined regimen to be worth the increased cost.[5]

The concept of cost-effectiveness is most meaningful when used in a relative manner. In other words, instead of addressing the cost-effectiveness of drug A alone, we examine the cost-effectiveness of drug A compared with drugs B and C. For example, if drug X is associated with costs of $10 000 for every life it saves, is it cost-effective? The answer depends on the subjective value system of the decision-maker. On the other hand, if it can be said that drug A has lower costs and equal or greater effectiveness as drug B, we can objectively say that drug A is the more cost-effective alternative. Of course, this comparison of alternative interventions does not ensure objectively interpretable results. For example, what if drug A is found both more costly and more effective than its al-

Table 1. Costs and Effectiveness of Drug A Compared with Drug B

Costs of Drug A	Effectiveness of Drug A	
	Higher than Drug B	Lower than Drug B
Higher than Drug B	X_1	X_2
Lower than Drug B	X_3	X_4

ternatives (e.g., cell X_1 of Table 1)? In this case, the need for value judgment is apparent and the decision cannot be entirely objective. Note, however, that even in this latter case in which the decision is more subjective, the information about costs and effectiveness of the other alternatives will lead to a more informed decision than if only the costs and effectiveness of drug A had been considered.

Thus, it is generally preferable to consider cost-effectiveness in this relative manner. There are two exceptions when comparison of alternatives may not be necessary: (1) when the only alternative available is the absence of the intervention in question, and (2) when the decision is obvious (i.e., virtually everyone concurs that the benefits gained are worth the cost). However, CEA rarely is conducted in such obvious situations as the latter where the use of formal decision techniques are not needed.

Principles of CEA

Warner and Luce[3] and Dao[4] have outlined the basic steps that apply to all CEA settings. Although they may seem obvious, failure to follow these steps has been detrimental to many analyses.[12] These steps are outlined in Figure 1 and discussed individually, with special references to drug therapy considerations.

DEFINING THE PROBLEM

There are three steps to problem definition. A prerequisite for successful CEA is that the analyst understand the point of view or perspective from which the analysis is to be conducted. The next step is to state the basic problem being addressed. Third, specific objectives should be selected against which the alternative interventions are to be evaluated.

Perspective. Different decision-makers have legitimate differences in perspective that can affect what should be included in the analysis. A societal perspective (the aggregate of all society members, present and future) requires that all direct and indirect costs be addressed, as well as direct and indirect benefits and all intangible effects, whether measurable or not. Through the concept of net costs, the framework of CEA allows for the explicit inclusion (i.e., in monetary measurement) of direct costs and benefits, as well as indirect costs and benefits (although the latter have not traditionally been incorporated explicitly in drug therapy CEAs). The intangible costs of an intervention (e.g., pain, suffering) are typically dealt with qualitatively in CEA as they are in CBA.

Perspectives that are more narrow than that of society include the hospital, the insurer, and the patient. Because they are narrower in scope, it is logical that these perspectives might not consider some costs and benefits important to society as a whole. Patients are concerned with costs only to the extent that the individual is responsible for payment. The insured individual pays only when there are deductibles, co-insurance, and limits on coverage. These are often only a small portion of the total costs. The individual patient, however, is extremely concerned with risks of productivity losses, morbidity, mortality, and QOL. The hospital, on the other hand, is concerned only with costs prior to discharge so that effects on patient productivity and rehabilitation costs are not included. From the perspective of the insurer, only those costs within the scope of coverage are relevant. As a result, conflicting decisions may arise from analyses conducted from differing perspectives.

Deciding which perspective to use is not always straightforward. The conventional view is to take the societal perspective, since the goals of CEA historically have been to determine what society should do with regard to resource allocation. However, this may not accurately reflect the primary concerns of a given patient, hospital, or insurer. A more narrow view is to accept that the proper perspective is that of the individual or organization for whom the analysis is being conducted. The latter approach often is too restrictive since, regardless of the point of view of the decision-maker for whom the analysis is being conducted,

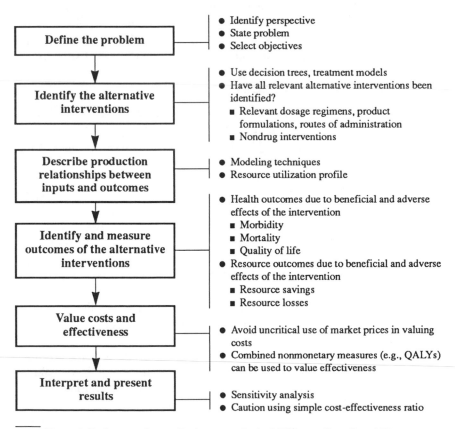

Figure 1. Basic steps of cost-effectiveness analysis. QALY = quality-adjusted life years.

it is likely that they will need to know how others will assess the situation. Policy recommendations will have to be adopted, implemented, enforced, and perhaps withstand litigation by agencies, institutions, and individuals who have their own perspectives. One solution to the dilemma is to provide modules or subanalyses that reflect the perspectives of the various interested parties.[4] Luft further expanded on this notion and suggested weighting the various subanalyses by the influence each group has in the decision-making process.[13] This would allow the analyst to predict what would happen given the power distribution of interested parties. Regardless of the approach taken, the decision regarding the perspectives to be taken must be made prior to beginning the CEA.

Perception of the Problem. The real starting point of the analysis is in identifying the problem. Traditional healthcare CEAs have started with a specific health problem (e.g., morbidity, disability, mortality) associated with a certain disease. Analysts then are motivated to identify and compare a wide variety of preventive and therapeutic modalities with respect to relative cost-effectiveness. More recently, a specific intervention strategy (e.g., a specific drug, surgical procedure, or piece of equipment) often has served as the starting point. The problem to be solved is whether the intervention in question, say drug X, is cost-effective rather than to determine the most cost-effective alternative for reducing morbidity and/or mortality from a particular condition. CEAs of drug therapy typically have reflected this type of problem orientation.[6,14-17] Because the analyst begins with a given pharmaceutical intervention in mind, the drug(s) in question can be studied for single or multiple conditions.

Although both problem orientations are legitimate and can arrive at identical CEAs, the latter orientation carries a risk of missing the forest for the trees.[3] For example, orientation toward comparative cost-effectiveness of cefaclor with amoxicillin for the treatment of acute otitis media might cause the analyst to overlook the fact that other drugs, such as amoxicillin/clavulanate or trimethoprim/ sulfamethoxazole, are reasonable alternatives that should be investigated simultaneously. More generally, orientation toward comparative cost-effectiveness of drug X with other drugs in its class might cause the analyst to overlook the possibility that some other drug, no treatment, nondrug treatment, or a preventive approach to the condition are reasonable alternatives that could be investigated simultaneously. In other words, it does not matter that drug X is more cost-effective than drug Y if another approach is better than both!

Thus, in conducting CEA of drug therapy, the analyst always must contemplate the implications of his problem orientation. If the problem is formulated in terms of a specific drug or drug class, consideration should be given to the documentation in the medical literature of the acceptability of alternatives to the drug(s) in question. It is quite proper to focus on drug-drug comparisons if the condition in question is known to require drug therapy. An example of the latter situation is illustrated by a CEA of alternative drug therapy approaches for long-term treatment of proximal venous thrombosis.[16]

Selection of Objectives. Specific objectives are selected next for comparing the effectiveness of alternative interventions. In other words, a decision must be made about how effectiveness will be evaluated. The previously established perspective of the analysis and problem statement will have laid the groundwork for this decision.

Selection of an appropriate, measurable objective (or objectives) is not always easy. Careful attention must be paid to the link between the health problem in question and the specific objective. Warner and Luce have used the example of morbidity and mortality due to myocardial infarction (MI) in order to illustrate the importance of this phase of CEA.[3] Both morbidity and mortality due to MI clearly are important aspects of the health problem. Approaches to reducing the problem would vary depending on which of the two objectives the analyst selects: decreasing the mortality rate of MI sufferers versus reducing the incidence of MIs. The first objective would suggest a variety of emergency treatment alternatives, whereas the latter suggests preventive approaches. The point is that selection of either objective does not allow consideration of intervention approaches suggested by the other. That is, preventive efforts would be expected to have little impact on mortality rates in patients with MIs and emergency treatment interventions would have little effect on the incidence.

In the above example, a dilemma exists. Whenever such a seeming incompatibility of possible objectives exists, the analyst has three choices: (1) to select one objective, thereby reducing the scope of the analysis; (2) to include both objectives, realizing the resulting analysis may be inconclusive due to the lack of a common unit of measure; or (3) to identify some other measurable objective that incorporates both concerns. In other words, to reiterate from the introductory discussion about the CEA framework, the analyst may choose to measure effectiveness with a single measure, multiple measures, or a combined measure. In the case of MIs, a reasonable solution might be to select quality-adjusted years of life as an objective. Both preventive and treatment approaches are consistent with this measure.

An example of the difficulties involved in selecting objectives is fairly specific to drug formulary decisions. Gagnon and Osterhaus have described in detail the aspects of CEA as they apply to formulary decision-making.[18] In such situations, the pharmacy and therapeutics committee typically considers the addition, deletion, or restricted use of a particular drug. Thus, the problem orientation is intervention- rather than health problem-based. Most drugs are used for more than one indication, and each indication may have different relevant health outcomes. Since a decision to add, delete, or restrict the use of a drug must consider all its potential uses, the pharmacy and therapeutics committee does not have the option of selecting a single measure from several seemingly incompatible measures. Either multiple objectives or some combined objectives must be identified.

In order to ensure the appropriateness of the selected objectives, the analyst should feel confident that the objectives chosen reflect the most important dimensions of the health problems and are relevant to the alternative interventions that will be compared. Furthermore, a measure should be selected that is sensitive to the actual differences likely to be encountered between interventions. For example, if the percent of patients cured with alternative drug regimens is expected to be similar, but time to healing or symptom resolution or recurrence rates are expected to differ, an objective reflecting the latter measures should be selected.

IDENTIFYING THE ALTERNATIVES

A well-defined problem and concrete objectives provide boundaries on the variety of alternative means of attacking the problem. In general, the narrower the problem and objectives, the fewer relevant alternatives there will be. For example, if the problem is the consequences of ulcer disease, all alternatives must be directed at those consequences. If the objective is to increase the healing rates of patients with active ulcers, preventive alternatives would be excluded.

Treatment models or decision trees describing possible diagnostic and therapeutic events for each disease are essential for identifying alternative interventions. Dao has demonstrated the use of treatment models in identifying alternative therapies for open-angle glaucoma.[4] Decision trees are much the same as treatment models, but have been adapted to suit the goals of decision analysis. The construction of decision trees is considered in detail in Chapter 7. A treatment model or decision tree diagrams the interventions available to patients with a specific disease and the flow of possible events resulting from the initial choice of intervention. These models or decision trees are constructed based on the medical literature concerning options for intervention. Figure 2 is an example of a decision tree depicting the alternative interventions and possible flow of events for a patient with a positive test result for a hypothetical disease.

In drug therapy CEAs, several types of interventions might be compared. In the simplest case, individual drugs may be compared for a single condition. The drugs in question do not necessarily have to be from different drug classes, but they usually are different with respect to some relevant pharmacologic property. For example, Holloway et al. compared the cost-effectiveness of gentamicin and tobramycin based on the premise that gentamicin has greater nephrotoxic potential.[15]

Interventions being compared also may be different classes of drugs (e.g., beta-blockers versus thiazide diuretics for the initial treatment of hypertension). When classes of drugs are compared, a single drug from each class often is selected as a representative for that class.

Interventions may be compared across multiple disease conditions, which is required for many formulary decisions.[18] For example, the histamine H_2-blockers cimetidine, ranitidine, and famotidine might be compared for both treatment of existing ulcers and prophylaxis of recurrent ulcers.

Depending on the scope of the problem and specific objectives being addressed, it may be necessary to include nondrug therapy (e.g., surgery) or even no therapy as alternative interventions. For example, in a CEA of isoniazid for tuberculosis prevention, the policy of avoiding drug therapy among older tuberculin reactors, who are at low risk for activation, has been evaluated.[19]

Other types of alternative interventions seen in the drug CEA literature include: single versus combination drug therapy (e.g., combined tetracycline and ampicillin versus either drug alone for endocervical gonorrhea),[14] drug therapy alone versus drug therapy plus other diagnostic or therapeutic modalities,[10,14] inpatient versus outpatient drug therapy,[20] alternative formulations of the same drug (e.g., premixed admixtures versus compounded doses),[21] and different dosage regimens of the same drug.[16] With all of these alternatives, however, it should be recognized that during the course of treatment these interventions are not mutually exclusive. For example, a patient with acute otitis media may fail to im-

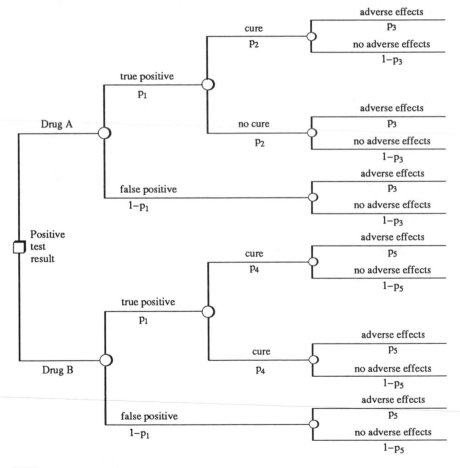

Figure 2. Decision tree demonstrating choices of action in a patient with a positive test result.

prove on the initial antibiotic selected (e.g., amoxicillin) and will require another antibiotic (e.g., cefaclor). Thus, when we identify amoxicillin or cefaclor as an alternative therapy, we are referring to the initial choice of antibiotics.

The most common pitfall in identifying alternatives arises when the analyst jumps directly to this stage of the analysis without having carefully defined the problem and objectives of the study. Under such circumstances, it is easy to identify the wrong alternatives. For example, an analyst might be interested at the outset in showing that a single dose of a new antibiotic is more cost-effective in surgical prophylaxis than multiple doses of an older antibiotic. Thus, these are the interventions identified for analysis. However, if the analyst had stepped back and really thought about the problem objectively (reducing postsurgical infection), it would have been obvious that these were the wrong alternatives to compare. The problem with the alternatives originally identified is that an even more relevant alternative is neglected—a single dose of the older (and less expensive) drug may be just as effective as the new antibiotic. As a consequence, the results of the CEA would have little practical use since it would not compare regimens that are appropriate for the problem in question.

DESCRIBING THE PRODUCTION RELATIONSHIPS

Defining the health problem, objectives, and alternatives establishes the conceptual framework of a CEA. The next step in the analysis—describing the relationship between resource inputs (production costs), resource outcomes (induced savings and losses), and health outcomes—expands upon this framework. Describing the production relationship ultimately results in identification and measurement of resources required to provide each intervention. It also provides the technical framework for the quantitative assessment and comparison of net costs with net effectiveness.

There are several methods for characterizing these production relationships. All approaches involve development of a model specifying how inputs are combined and how much output a given grouping of inputs will produce. An important aspect of these models is the assessment of marginal inputs and outputs. In brief, the tendency of many analysts is to rely on average inputs needed to produce a unit of output. There are several problems with this approach, among which is the overestimation of opportunity costs of an intervention by inclusion of its associated fixed inputs. The appropriate approach is to address the question: For each additional unit of input, how much additional output will be gained? This concept of marginal analysis has been discussed in detail in Chapter 3.

The model may be as simple as a flow chart, identifying all inputs and their quantities at the points where they enter the production process, or it may be a more complicated technique. Modeling techniques that can be used include: Monte Carlo and Markov Chain models, decision analysis, and linear programming. Decision analysis has been the most commonly employed modeling technique in drug therapy CEAs.[5,6,10,14,15]

Use of Decision Analysis. We briefly introduced the concept of decision analysis when we described decision trees to be used for identifying alternative interventions. As described above, the structure of the decision tree diagrams possible flows of events resulting from the different interventions (decisions). The underlying decision tree structure is all that has been necessary until this point. However, there are two additions to the structure of the decision tree that must be made in order to determine the production relationship. First, it becomes necessary to add probabilities of the various events to the tree (see Chapter 7 for details). Given the fact that a therapy usually produces more than one health outcome, and that few outcomes occur in 100 percent of patients, estimates of probabilities with which a given event occurs are needed. These probabilities then are inserted into the decision tree. Thus, in Figure 2, regardless of the intervention (drug A versus drug B), there is a probability, p_1, that the positive test result will be a true positive and a probability, $1-p_1$, that it will be a false positive result. Since these values will influence whether the drug will be effective (a health outcome), they must be included in the production relationship. Further along the decision tree, drug A can produce four outcomes: cure (p_2), no cure ($1-p_2$), adverse effects (p_3), and no adverse effects ($1-p_3$). The decision tree and its attached probabilities provide the technical framework for calculating how much of a given outcome (e.g., number of cures per 100 persons treated with drug A) can be expected with each intervention.

To complete the modeling process, a resource utilization profile is developed that parallels the structure of the decision tree, but delineates all health resources involved in each step of the decision tree.

The Resource Utilization Profile. For each event represented in the corresponding decision tree, the use of such health resources as services by physicians and other health professionals, hospital services, diagnostic tests, and drug therapy must be identified. This information must be specific, detailing the exact quantities and types of resources needed. For services by professionals, the specific services and the type of professional providing them must be specified. Is the service provided by a physician, nurse, or pharmacist? Even more specifically, how specialized are these professionals? Is the nurse an L.P.N., an R.N., or a nurse practitioner? One particular service provided by nurses that is especially relevant to drug therapy CEAs is drug administration. For pharmacists, the time involved in traditional dispensing services (e.g., compounding, supervision of technicians) as well as any progressive pharmacy service (e.g., pharmacokinetic monitoring) that are a part of the particular intervention should be itemized. The number of times each service is provided by each of these professionals and the time required per episode is also required. For hospital services, the type of unit on which the services are provided should be specified (e.g., intensive care unit, burn unit, emergency room). Furthermore, the number of days or hours spent in each type of unit is needed. Specific diagnostic tests and the number of times each is employed must be identified. For drug therapy, the analyst must specify the specific drugs, their dose, dosing interval, duration of therapy, and route of administration. The health resources discussed so far have all been direct production costs. As discussed at the beginning of this chapter, indirect production costs— resources used indirectly in the production process—may also be included, depending on the perspective of the analysis. An example of the latter is the amount of patient time required to participate in the intervention.

Once probabilities have been inserted into the decision tree, the resource utilization profile has been completed and the production relationship has been completely described. The resource utilization profile allows us to calculate total production costs required by each intervention.

IDENTIFYING AND MEASURING OUTCOMES OF EACH INTERVENTION

There are two types of outcomes that result from an intervention: health and resource outcomes. Health outcomes refer to changes in morbidity, mortality, and QOL, whereas resource outcomes refer to induced resource savings on avoided costs of illness and induced resource losses due to adverse effects of the intervention. Resource outcomes (induced savings and losses) are distinguished from resource use (production costs) in that the latter are limited to resources employed to produce the identified outcomes.

Analytically, measurement of health and resource outcomes often is performed indirectly by comparing with a no-therapy alternative. In other words, differences in the magnitude of outcomes would first be measured between each intervention and no therapy. Then, the different interventions would be compared in terms of their relative savings and losses against the no-therapy alternative. For example, if both drug A and B are used to prevent coronary heart disease, the health and resource outcomes with drug A would be compared with no therapy at all, and likewise for drug B. One reason for this practice is that this is the way data are typically available (i.e., many drug efficacy studies compare a drug with placebo).

IDENTIFYING AND MEASURING HEALTH OUTCOMES

If the problem, objectives, and alternative interventions have been carefully developed, identification of relevant health outcomes already will have been accomplished. In fact, these must be identified in order to complete the decision trees linking inputs to outcomes. Health outcomes may occur as a result of both the beneficial and adverse effects of an intervention.

Probabilities of the various events that may result from an intervention (e.g., of cure, adverse reactions, or death) will have been incorporated into these decision trees in the course of defining the production relationship. These probabilities are instrumental in measuring health outcomes.

Sources of Data About Health Outcomes. The actual values for the probabilities in the various branches of the decision tree can be obtained from a wide variety of sources, including primary data collection by the analyst. The clinical literature and expert opinion are other sources.

Estimates of required probabilities often are based on results of multiple studies of a similar topic. In order to derive a single probability estimate from these multiple sources, meta-analysis can be used. Cochran's method of meta-analysis, which pools results by assigning weights to different studies to reflect their sample sizes and the similarity of their results,[22] was used by Weinstein et al. to estimate aminoglycoside toxicity rates. A search was conducted of articles published since 1969 in English-language journals, and data from the papers found to meet minimal criteria of study design were combined using meta-analysis.[5]

Critical Evaluation of Published Literature. Careful and discriminatory evaluation of published studies is essential to avoiding misinterpretation of study results. Polk and Hepler reviewed the problems with design and statistical evaluation of clinical trials and made recommendations for evaluating study outcomes.[23] A common conclusion of a randomized trial is that there is no significant difference between the two regimens being compared. In fact, many drug therapy CEAs are based upon such studies. Thus, an analyst will assume equal health effectiveness of two interventions and proceed to conduct a comparative cost analysis, concluding that the intervention with the lowest cost is, therefore, most cost-effective.

When a study reports that two therapies are equivalent, there are actually three possible reasons why no significant difference was found.[22] First, the conclusion may be correct. This may be a proper interpretation if the sample size was sufficient and the differences in outcome are clinically unimportant. However, a conclusion of equivalence may be reached even if there is a real difference between the two regimens. Such a difference may not be detected in a study for two reasons: (1) the study lacked sufficient power to detect clinically important differences (type II error), or (2) there are confounding factors or a flawed study design obscuring the difference. The likelihood of a type II error is higher when the sample size is small and differences are described between groups that could be clinically important. When two regimens are compared and both are expected to be highly effective, it is especially difficult to demonstrate that one regimen is better than the other. This is because the difference between the two, even if clinically meaningful, is likely to be small and the sample size required to achieve statistical significance may be quite large. Tables are available for estimating the probability that a clinically important difference was missed in a study because of insufficient sample size.[24]

Similarly, when a study reports that one regimen is significantly superior to another, there are three possible explanations for the finding. First, the author's conclusion may be correct. This is most likely when the observed differences are clinically important. However, there may be no real difference between regimens in spite of detecting a significant difference. There are two reasons that this can happen: (1) the difference was due to a type I error; in other words, the probability of finding a difference when there is actually no difference; or (2) confounding factors or poor study design produced an artificial difference. The best protection against committing a type I error is to seek independent confirmation of the finding (i.e., through multiple studies). Thus, one should treat a conclusion of unequivalent effects in a single study as tentative, even if the study is well-designed, until independent confirmation can be made from the results of other studies. In summary, when conducting a CEA, the analyst must be as cautious in accepting the conclusion of differences between regimens as in accepting the conclusion of no difference. Either error can have tremendous impact on the resulting analysis.

The Randomized Controlled Trial: Efficacy versus Effectiveness. The majority of drug studies are randomized controlled trials (RCT). Since RCTs occur under ideal conditions, it is unreasonable to expect that the probabilities (e.g., of drug efficacy) obtained from them will be representative of what can be expected when drugs are used under less than ideal conditions, i.e., in the "real world." Thus, it is desirable to distinguish between the concepts of efficacy (how well the drug works under ideal conditions) and effectiveness (how well it works under conditions of average use). Unfortunately, whereas estimates of drug efficacy are relatively easy to come by, estimates of effectiveness are not. However, results from RCTs can be used (i.e., drug efficacy) and adjustments made to reflect expected conditions of actual use, such as diagnostic inaccuracies and alterations in drug intake due to prescriber and patient noncompliance with recommended regimens. These adjustments are often subjective in nature, since few data are available for most drugs regarding the relationship between degree of compliance and drug effect. The Lipid Research Clinics-Coronary Primary Prevention Trial (LRC-CPPT) is an example of a rare study able to quantify the relationship between patient compliance and drug effect.[25] A recent CEA of antihyperlipemic therapy in the prevention of coronary heart disease was able to use this observed relationship to estimate both the expected degree of compliance with recommended regimens and the fractional reduction in drug efficacy that would result.[2]

Other Sources of Health Outcome Data. Observational studies are other sources of data about health outcomes. These studies provide information on the strength of associations between certain factors (e.g., intervention, patient age, patient smoking history) and occurrence of disease or disease outcome. These studies may be either retrospective or prospective, but usually lack the random allocation of subjects seen with RCTs. They offer an advantage in that they may more accurately reflect conditions of actual drug use outside the ideal conditions of the RCT. The Hypertension Detection and Follow-Up Program is one of the better known studies of this type.[26]

Information required to estimate the decision tree probabilities is sometimes not at all available in the medical literature . Other times, the data available are scant and their reliability questionable. Under such circumstances, probabilities may be arrived at by obtaining the judgments of panels of physicians based on their clinical experience.

Until recently, health outcomes typically have been expressed in terms of morbidity and mortality rates associated with a disease or intervention. However, much emphasis has been placed in recent years on improving the QOL.[8,27] Since many current interventions, especially drug regimens, are aimed at alleviating disease conditions or relieving symptoms rather than at saving lives, the ability to measure QOL is important. Because this is a relatively new area of research, much controversy exists regarding the best methods for measuring QOL effects, but the consensus is that these methods are definitely feasible and highly desirable.[26] Even if the analyst chooses not to measure QOL as a health outcome, it should be at least dealt with descriptively in the presentation of the results.

IDENTIFYING AND MEASURING RESOURCE OUTCOMES

As with health outcomes, resource outcomes derive both from the beneficial and adverse effects of an intervention. Resource outcomes are the induced losses and savings associated with an intervention. Beneficial effects result in resource savings (induced savings), whereas adverse effects result in resource losses (induced losses). Both resource savings and losses can be either direct or indirect effects of the intervention in question.

Direct health resource savings refer to savings on direct medical costs of illness that would occur if the intervention were not present. Direct medical costs of illness are defined and illustrated in Chapter 3. For example, in a CEA of antihyperlipemic therapy in the prevention of coronary heart disease, the direct health resource savings associated with the intervention (antihyperlipemic therapy) would be the expected savings in lifetime medical care costs as a result of a decreased incidence of coronary heart disease.[2]

Direct health resource losses are direct medical costs associated with the adverse effects of an intervention, including the costs of diagnosing and treating adverse effects. In the above example, the direct health resource losses associated with antihyperlipemic therapy would be the expected cost of treating medication-related adverse effects over the course of therapy.

As discussed previously, indirect resource savings and losses also can be included in a CEA, depending on the perspective of the analysis. Illness can affect both the time people work and their productivity while working, in order to affect overall work output. Indirect resource outcomes thus occur in the form of work productivity savings (e.g., due to avoided illness) and losses (e. g., due to adverse effects). Savings and losses in time spent by patients and families receiving medical care are other types of resource outcome.

===== **VALUING COSTS AND EFFECTIVENESS**

Much has already been said in this and previous chapters about valuing effectiveness and costs, respectively, and is briefly summarized here.

Valuation of Costs. The valuation of economic costs entails conversion of production resource use, induced savings, and induced losses (measured in quantities of resources) into dollar value. This process has been discussed in detail in Chapter 3 but one important point will be reiterated here: uncritical use of market prices should be avoided since there are times when they may not reflect the true opportunity costs of resources (e.g., use of hospital charges to reflect cost of hospital care). It should be mentioned, however, that, although adjustment of market prices to represent true opportunity cost is important from a societal perspective, charges may be more relevant to analyses from an insurer's standpoint.

In spite of the above discussion, market prices of outpatient drugs generally are considered to reflect true opportunity costs much more closely than prices of nondrug health services. This is because the vast majority of outpatient prescriptions are paid for with out-of-pocket money.

Valuation of Effectiveness. The effectiveness of an intervention is not valued in monetary units. Many CEAs avoid this valuation altogether and simply provide rates of various health outcomes for each intervention (e.g., mortality rates, cure rates, rates of adverse reactions). However, when there is more than one relevant health effect, it may be desirable to use some nonmonetary valuation method in order to provide a single unit of measure. Such combined effectiveness measures were described in this chapter's introductory discussion of the CEA framework. Examples of methods for nonmonetary valuation of health effectiveness include the QALY[7] and utility analysis.[10] The QALY method has been the most extensively employed of these methods; however, we have mentioned the inherent difficulties involved in adjusting for QOL with this approach.

Discounting Costs and Effectiveness. Even if all costs, present and future, are adjusted for inflation, it is still necessary to discount future costs. The reason is that a dollar not spent now can be invested to yield a larger number of dollars in the future. The need to discount costs is unquestioned—only the choice of a discount rate is somewhat controversial. This and relevant issues have been discussed in Chapter 3.

Although the need to discount costs is accepted, some controversy remains regarding the need to discount nonmonetary effectiveness. Some researchers advocate discounting effectiveness because people generally prefer to have additional life years sooner than later. These proponents further state that a sufficient reason to discount effectiveness is that it is being valued relative to discounted costs.[1] Those who disagree state that there is no trade-off between having additional life years sooner than later, since you cannot have them later if you do not have them sooner.[4] Most healthcare CEAs that have discounted costs have also discounted effectiveness.

INTERPRETATION AND PRESENTATION OF RESULTS

Once costs and effectiveness of alternative interventions are identified, measured, valued, and discounted, the results of the analysis must be interpreted and presented in usable form. This phase of the analysis includes sensitivity analysis of uncertain assumptions, which has been described in previous chapters.

Since many of the estimates employed in CEA are uncertain, there is a strong need to test the sensitivity of the results to changes in these estimates. If the results of the analysis change little when these estimates are varied, confidence in the results is increased. On the other hand, if the results change substantially, then the analyst should be more concerned about the uncertainty of the particular estimate. Common sources of uncertainty are efficacy rates (especially comparative efficacy of the alternative interventions), adverse reaction rates, event rates in untreated individuals, estimates of cost components, and the selected discount rate. A useful approach to sensitivity analysis is the establishment of confidence intervals around the various estimates and then allowing the estimates to take on the upper and lower bounds of the interval. This is especially useful when the results of multiple studies provide varying estimates, since these multiple estimates can aid in establishing reasonable upper and lower bounds.

Extreme caution in interpretation and, ultimately, presentation of the results of the CEA is important. Readers of CEAs will rely heavily on the analyst's interpretation since the reader usually is privy only to the presented summary of the analysis. The presentation of results should clearly identify the critical uncertainties of the analysis along with discussion of the likely impact of these uncertainties on the results of the analysis. Furthermore, any relevant considerations that have not been addressed in the analysis should be discussed. For example, if health outcomes such as changes in QOL were identified but not addressed quantitatively, these should be discussed along with their likely impact on the analysis.

Even the manner in which the results are displayed must be given serious consideration. The temptation is to rely solely on the cost-effectiveness ratio as an index of the relative merit of the alternative interventions. Using this ratio as a criterion, the most cost-effective intervention would be the one with the lowest cost per unit effectiveness. However, this ratio should not be used uncritically. Under certain circumstances, the cost-effectiveness ratio will be misleading. The following example illustrates a situation where the cost-effectiveness ratio is deceptive. Suppose the cost-effectiveness of drug A is compared with that of drug B. Drug A results in a QALY savings (over no treatment) of ten QALYs at a cost of $1500. Drug B costs $3000, but will save 15 QALYs. The cost-effectiveness ratio of drug A is $150 per QALY saved which is superior to $200 per QALY saved for drug B. Thus, according to the simple cost-effectiveness ratio criterion, drug A is the best alternative since it costs the least per QALY saved. Yet few decision-makers would choose drug A over drug B, because the incremental cost-effectiveness ratio for drug B compared with drug A is ($3000–$1500) / (15–10) = $300 per QALY gained by choosing drug B over drug A—presumably a worthwhile investment!

Thus, whenever one or more alternative interventions both costs more and is more effective, the simple cost-effectiveness ratio can be misleading. Under such circumstances, greater insight would be provided by analyzing incremental cost-effectiveness ratios as above. Another alternative is to characterize the alternative interventions in terms of their costs and effectiveness without converting them into ratios.[3]

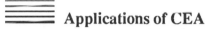 ## Applications of CEA

The application of CEA techniques is illustrated in the following three case studies. Each is derived from an actual CEA publication in the clinical literature. The accompanying critical appraisals of each study are intended to emphasize important CEA issues and not to criticize the studies themselves. In fact, all three studies were selected because of their overall high quality.

CASE STUDY NO. 1: ANTIBIOTIC PROPHYLAXIS OF CESAREAN SECTION

The results of a cost-effectiveness comparison of cefonicid sodium versus cefoxitin sodium for the prevention of postoperative infections after nonelective cesarean section have been published. Using a double-blind, randomized, controlled trial design, 60 women received cefonicid 1 g iv at cord clamping followed by two iv placebo doses, and another 60 women received cefoxitin 2 g iv at cord clamping followed by two similar doses at six-hour intervals. The outcomes measured were febrile morbidity (defined as an oral temperature $\geq$100.4 °F occurring twice, at least six hours apart, within the first ten postpartum days, excluding the first 24 hours) and occurrence of documented infections. Three types of infections were considered: endometritis, wound infection, and urinary tract infection. No significant differences in patient demographic characteristics or in risk factors for postoperative infection were found between the two groups. No significant differences were found between groups in occurrences of febrile morbidity or rates of documented infections. Adverse reactions occurred in only two patients. The only costs measured were drug acquisition costs. The difference between the acquisition cost for three doses of cefoxitin and one dose of cefonicid for 838 cesarean sections per year was estimated to be $29 975. The authors concluded that, in the dosage regimens used, cefonicid is more cost-effective than cefoxitin for preventing post-cesarean section infectious morbidity.[28]

Critique. The implied perspective of the analysis is that of the hospital. The authors perceived that the problem to be addressed was whether single-dose therapy would be more cost-effective than multiple-dose therapy. The objective of the study was clear: to prevent postoperative infections.

The authors' single- versus multiple-dose orientation when approaching the problem may have caused them to fail to identify relevant alternatives for analysis. If they really were interested in discovering the most cost-effective approach to antibiotic prophylaxis of cesarean section, other possible regimens might have been found even better if studied. Other alternatives that might have been included would be an older (therefore, less expensive) accepted drug in a multiple-dose regimen, single-dose cefoxitin, or any of a group of other antibiotics that are used in this therapeutic situation.

The only production cost identified and measured was drug acquisition. Although the authors identified nursing and pharmacy time as relevant concerns, neither were measured and included as production costs.

Identification and measurement of most health outcomes was excellent. Since few adverse reactions were identified, they were assumed to occur equally between groups and were not included in the CEA. Similarly, since the two regimens appeared to be equal in efficacy and adverse effects, it was assumed that no resource savings or resource losses would be induced for either regimen. The major problem with these assumptions of equal efficacy and adverse effects is that, although none of the differences between the two groups were significant, the power of the study to detect a clinically meaningful halving of the infection rate was only 35 percent. To achieve 90 percent power, roughly 250 subjects per group would be required. If, in fact, differences did exist between the groups in efficacy and/or adverse effects, the difference between groups in associated resource savings and losses could no longer be assumed to be zero.

The authors chose to present multiple effectiveness measures rather than attempt to use a combined measure. Neither costs nor effectiveness was discounted. This probably was appropriate since this was an acute situation in which neither costs nor benefits are likely to occur over a long period of time following therapy.

The uncertainty of various assumptions made in the analysis was not addressed. Assumptions that could have been subjected to sensitivity analysis were the assumptions of equal efficacy and adverse effects, which could be criticized because of low study power. In presenting their results, the authors did mention the possibility of a type II error; however, they failed to discuss the implications of this for their analysis. One might justify the assumption of equal efficacy by saying that if a real difference in efficacy existed, it is likely to be in favor of cefonicid. In that case, the study results would not be changed; rather, the relative efficacy of cefonicid and, hence, associated resource savings would have been underestimated under this study's assumptions. This may be a reasonable argument since, although not statistically significant, the rates of all types of infectious morbidity were lower in the cefonicid group. The same argument cannot be made for adverse effects since the data are much too scarce.

A similar argument could be used for including only drug acquisition costs as production costs. Since the cefoxitin regimen requires multiple doses, associated compounding and administration costs would be higher for that regimen. Thus, the study underestimates the production costs associated with cefoxitin, and inclusion of these other components would only increase the relative cost-effectiveness of the cefonicid regimen. The authors did not discuss these issues.

The authors concluded that, since efficacy and toxicity were demonstrated to be equivalent, the decision to select one antibiotic over the other should be based on cost. Since cefonicid was the least costly, it is, therefore, most cost-effective. These are valid conclusions but, because they rely on the assumptions of equal efficacy and toxicity, the authors should have discussed the potential effects of violating these assumptions.

CASE STUDY NO. 2: TOPICAL VERSUS SYSTEMIC ACNE TREATMENT

Cost-effectiveness analysis was used to compare two strategies for clearing papulopustular acne: topical therapy alone as initial therapy or initial treatment with a combination of systemic antibiotics and topical agents. Each strategy was displayed in the form of a decision tree. Although the topical agent strategy initiates therapy with topical agents only, the decision tree allowed for those patients who failed on this regimen to be switched later to systemic therapy. As is common in CEA studies, no actual patients were involved in the study. Rather, two sources of data were used to determine the decision tree probabilities: the literature and a survey of dermatologists (the latter was used to obtain probability estimates when data were not available in the literature). Costs were estimated as physician visits plus drug costs necessary to achieve clearing of the acne. The outcomes assessed were weeks of morbidity from acne until clearing (or failure) and episodes of adverse effects. Clearing was defined as a decrease of at least 50 percent in lesion count or a good-to-excellent response based on clinical assessment.[6]

The systemic agent strategy had six fewer weeks of morbidity from acne per patient, lower costs of care (about $20 per patient), and twice the number of adverse effects as the topical agent strategy. When sensitivity analysis was conducted, the magnitude of these differences changed, but the direction of the differences did not. The choice of topical therapy in a population of patients was estimated to cost an additional $764 to avoid one additional episode of adverse effects (most commonly gastrointestinal upset and vaginitis). Choice of the topical therapy would also cost an additional 4.6 years of morbidity (since topical therapy is less efficacious in achieving clearing) to avert one additional episode of adverse effects. The authors judged that neither price would be worth paying to reduce the risk of adverse effects and concluded that initial treatment with combined systemic antibiotics and topical agents was most cost-effective. The authors suggested that patients with an increased risk of vaginitis or gastrointestinal adverse effects, however, might be willing to accept a longer period of morbidity from acne in order to avoid the development of an adverse effect.[6]

Critique. The implied perspective of the analysis is that of the patient and of the physician as patient advocate. The authors perceived the problem as a clinical dilemma: they observed that the clinical literature advocates initial treatment with topical therapy alone, although practicing dermatologists frequently prescribe systemic agents as part of a patient's initial treatment regimen. Realizing that the use of systemic agents is associated with adverse drug effects that may add dollar costs, but also may save costs by speeding resolution and reducing the need for return visits, the authors' objectives were clear: to measure the time to clearing, the episodes of adverse drug effects, and the associated resource savings and losses.

The authors' orientation toward deciding which of two interventions should be preferred may have led them to omit another relevant regimen: systemic antibiotics alone. Such a strategy would have lower drug costs than the combined therapy and, if efficacy was not much less, the number of physician visits might be similar to that of the combined regimen.

The authors used the techniques of decision analysis to define the production relationship between production costs and health (and associated resource) outcomes. It appears that they have included relevant direct production costs (medication costs and physician visits). However, indirect production costs were not included. Since the perspective of the analysis was that of the patient, it would be reasonable to include the indirect costs of patient and family time involved in the treatment process. The specific dollar costs associated with each cost component were not itemized. This would have been helpful since, without this information, the reader is unable to evaluate the appropriateness of the estimated follow-up frequency (number of physician visits) and dollar values assigned to physician visits.

Relevant health and direct resource outcomes were identified and measured appropriately. Since the topical agent strategy allowed for adding systemic antibiotics for patients who fail to improve, there was no difference between strategies in number of patients who clear. Thus, since there was no difference in this health outcome, there was no associated induced resource savings for either intervention. However, the difference in rates of clearing is reflected within the production relationship and was associated with substantially lower production costs for the systemic strategy. Since the strategies had different rates of adverse reactions, there was an associated induced resource loss due to treatment of adverse effects (medication costs and physician visits). Indirect resource outcomes were not included. Since the implied perspective of the study was that of the patient, it would have been reasonable to include the indirect resources losses of patient and family time required for treatment of adverse effects.

Two effectiveness measures were employed (weeks of morbidity from acne and episodes of adverse effects per 1000 patients). Estimates of efficacy, adverse effect rates, and medication costs were displayed along with the ranges employed in the sensitivity analysis. As with the previous case study, neither costs nor effectiveness was discounted, which probably was appropriate due to the acute nature of the clinical question. One- and two-variable sensitivity analyses were conducted for all relevant variables. The presentation of results included a detailed discussion of the sensitivity analysis and implications for the study's conclusions. The authors acknowledged that their analysis was designed only to consider the relative costs and effectiveness up to the time a patient's condition clears or fails to clear. They recognized that acne is a chronic condition requiring maintenance therapy to keep a patient free of acne following clearing, but cost-effectiveness of alternative approaches of maintenance therapy was not within the scope of the study.

CASE STUDY NO. 3: ANTIHYPERLIPEMIC THERAPY
AND CORONARY HEART DISEASE

Using cholestyramine as a model, a study evaluated the cost-effectiveness of antihyperlipemic therapy in the primary prevention of coronary heart disease in men with elevated levels of total plasma cholesterol (≥265 mg/dL). The perspective adopted was societal. All data were obtained from the literature. The ratio of net change in medical care costs to the net increase in life expectancy was calculated:

$$C/E = (dCRx + dCSE - dCMorb + dCRxdLE) / dLE \qquad \text{Eq. 1}$$

where dCRx indicates the expected lifetime cost of drug therapy (based on a national survey of retail pharmacy prices for bulk cholestyramine); dCSE, the expected cost of treating medication-related adverse effects over the course of therapy; dCMorb, the expected savings in lifetime medical care costs as a result of a decreased incidence of cardiovascular disease; dCRxdLE, the expected cost of treating noncardiac diseases during the years of additional life conferred by treatment; and dLE, the increase in life expectancy resulting from adherence to a specified regimen of drug therapy. All future costs and changes in life expectancy were discounted at a rate of five percent. Baseline estimates of cost-effectiveness were calculated assuming a dosage of 16 g/d, which was the mean daily intake in the LRC-CPPT. The LRC-CPPT results also were used to determine the expected relationship between drug dose and decline in cholesterol level.[24]

A multivariate logistic function from the 16-year follow-up of Framingham Heart Study (FHS)[29] participants was used to estimate future annual probabilities of coronary heart disease (CHD) for patients with given risk factors, including cholesterol level and age. Future coronary risk was estimated for various age groups. To estimate the reduction in coronary risk due to treatment, the expected reduction in cholesterol from various initial concentrations were first calculated using LRC-CPPT data. The FHS logistic function was then used to estimate, for the different combinations of pre- and posttreatment levels, the maximum possible reduction in risk. The authors then assumed that patients would not benefit from treatment during the first two years—corresponding to the LRC-CPPT experience—but they would realize maximum possible benefit in succeeding years. These reductions in risk then were used to calculate changes in life expectancy and lifetime medical care costs as a result of therapy (dLE, dCMorb, and dCRxdLE). Cost-effectiveness was evaluated for varying lengths of therapy and for subgroups of patients defined by specific constellations of concomitant risk factors. Sensitivity analysis was conducted for several assumptions and parameter estimates.

Cost-effectiveness of lifelong therapy varied from $56 100 per year of life saved to over $1 million, depending on age at initiation of therapy and pretreatment cholesterol level. Costs per life-year gained were lower for younger patients and for those with higher pretreatment levels of cholesterol. Less-than-lifelong therapy generally was more cost-effective than lifelong therapy. The exception to this was that therapy lasting only a few years was less cost-effective than lifelong therapy, reflecting the assumed absence of benefit during the first two years of treatment. Cost-effectiveness varied according to concomitant risk factors, with cost per life-year gained declining as the number of coronary risk factors increases.

Critique. The societal perspective was stated clearly. The authors' problem orientation was toward weighing the economic cost of antihyperlipemic therapy against its clinical benefit. The objectives were to reduce the number of life-years lost due to CHD.

The perspective and objectives of the analysis were consistent with evaluation of a wide variety of alternative approaches to prevent or treat CHD and the authors evaluated only one of these. Other interventions to which cholesterol lowering might be compared are antihypertensive therapy, coronary bypass surgery, and beta-blockade in post-MI patients.[30] Since such a comprehensive analysis would be extremely time consuming, the authors focused on a single intervention. Thus, this study is useful from the standpoint of quantifying the expected costs and increased life expectancy due to cholesterol lowering and for assessing how the balance of costs and life-years saved varies according to duration of treatment and concomitant risk factors. It can be used only indirectly (through comparison with other cost-effectiveness studies) to assess the relative cost-effectiveness of cholesterol lowering compared with alternative interventions.

The production relationship was modeled using the dose/response relationship observed in the LRC-CPPT trial and a multivariate logistic function calibrated to the FHS. Direct resource use (dCRx) was evaluated appropriately using estimated retail price and expected mean daily drug intake. Indirect resource costs were not included although their inclusion would have been consistent with the societal perspective.

The health outcomes identified and measured were: (1) risk of coronary heart disease (measured as life expectancy), and (2) occurrence of gastrointestinal adverse effects. Associated direct resource outcomes were induced savings on expected lifetime medical care costs as a result of decreased incidence of cardiovascular disease (dCMorb), and induced losses resulting from treatment of adverse effects (dCSE), and treating noncardiac diseases that occur in added years of life (dCRxLE). Although it is controversial, it can be argued that inclusion of these costs occurring in added years of life overestimates the induced costs associated with antihyperlipemic therapy. Indirect resource savings and losses were not included.

Although the occurrence of adverse effects was measured, this information was used only in determining the induced resource losses due to their treatment. The occurrence of adverse effects was not included in the measure of net health effectiveness in spite of their likely effect on QOL. Effectiveness was measured as the increase in life expectancy that results from antihyperlipemic therapy. Both costs and effectiveness were appropriately discounted since both costs and changes in life expectancy were projected years into the future.

The interpretation and presentation of the results were extensive. Incremental cost-effectiveness of continuing treatment each additional five years was presented, expressed as the ratio of the increase in discounted cost of therapy divided by the resulting increase in life-years saved due to these additional years of treatment. Extensive discussion of the results of sensitivity analysis and their likely impact on the results of the analysis was provided. Finally, a complete presentation of the methodologic limitations of the study was included, with corresponding interpretation of their likely effects on the study results.

Summary

Cost-effectiveness analysis is a means of identifying, measuring, and comparing the net resources costs and net health effectiveness of alternative health-care practices. Net resource costs are calculated as production costs plus induced resource losses minus induced resource savings. Production costs are the resources used to actually provide an intervention. Induced resource losses are the resources consumed in tests and treatments undertaken as a consequence of the initial intervention. Induced resource savings are resource expenditures that are averted as a consequence of the initial intervention. Net health effectiveness includes the beneficial and adverse effects of an intervention and is measured using a nonmonetary approach. Single, combined, or multiple nonmonetary effectiveness measures can be used.

Cost-effectiveness is used to imply value for money. If a drug costs less and is more effective than another, it is clearly the most cost-effective of the two. However, when one drug both costs more and is more effective than another, the decision of relative cost-effectiveness depends on whether the decision-maker feels the extra effectiveness is worth the extra costs.

In conducting a CEA, the perspective of the analysis, a well-defined problem statement, and concrete objectives provide boundaries on the variety of alternative interventions. Decision trees or other modeling techniques are important for identifying alternative interventions and for describing the production relationship between resource inputs and resource and health outcomes. These outcomes can be measured by primary data collection, by obtaining information from published studies, or from expert opinion. Critical evaluation of published studies is important for obtaining accurate estimates of health and resource outcomes. Discounting should be used to measure future costs and effectiveness, and sensitivity analysis of important uncertainties should be conducted. The analyst's presentation and discussion of results is critical to appropriate interpretation by readers. Caution should be exercised when using the simple cost-effectiveness ratio to summarize results, since there are conditions under which this will be misleading. Incremental cost-effectiveness ratios or presenting costs and effectiveness without constructing ratios is preferred in these situations. Several examples illustrated these points and demonstrated the techniques of CEA.

References

1. Weinstein MC, Stason WB. Foundations of cost-effectiveness analysis for health and medical practices. *N Engl J Med* 1977;*296*:716-21.
2. Oster G, Epstein AM. Cost-effectiveness of antihyperlipemic therapy in the prevention of coronary heart disease: the case of cholestyramine. *JAMA* 1987;*258*:2381-7.
3. Warner KE, Luce BR. Cost-benefit and cost-effectiveness analysis in health care: principles, practice, and potential. Ann Arbor, MI: Health Administration Press, 1982.

4. Dao TD. Cost-benefit and cost-effectiveness analysis of drug therapy. *Am J Hosp Pharm* 1985;*42*:791-802.

5. Weinstein MC, Read JL, MacKay DN, et al. Cost-effective choice of antimicrobial therapy for serious infections. *J Gen Intern Med* 1986;*1*:351-63.

6. Stern RS, Pass RM, Komaroff AL. Topical versus systemic agent treatment for papulopustular acne: cost-effectiveness analysis. *Arch Dermatol* 1984;*120*:1571-8.

7. Weinstein MC, Fineberg HV. Clinical decision analysis. Philadelphia: WB Saunders, 1980:253-4.

8. Vinokur A. Application of quality of life and well-being measurement as input into cost-effectiveness analyses. *Drug Info J* 1988;*22*:311-6.

9. Croog SH, Levine S, Testa MA, et al. The effects of antihypertensive therapy on the quality of life. *N Engl J Med* 1986;*314*:1657-64.

10. Nettleman MD, Jones RB, Roberts SD, et al. Cost-effectiveness of culturing for *Chlamydia trachomatis*: a study in a clinic for sexually transmitted diseases. *Ann Intern Med* 1986;*105*:189-96.

11. Doubilet P, Weinstein MC, McNeil BJ. Use and misuse of the term "cost-effective" in medicine. *N Engl J Med* 1986;*314*:253-5.

12. Warner KE, Hutton R. Cost-benefit and cost-effectiveness analysis in health care: growth and composition of the literature. *Med Care* 1980;*18*:1069-84.

13. Luft HS. Benefit cost analysis and public policy implementation: from normative to positive analysis. *Public Policy* 1976;*24*:437-61.

14. Washington AE, Browner WS, Korenbrot CC. Cost-effectiveness of combined treatment for endocervical gonorrhea considering co-infection with *Chlamydia trachomatis*. *JAMA* 1987;*257*:2056-60.

15. Holloway JJ, Smith CR, Moor RD, Feroli ER, Lietman PS. Comparative cost-effectiveness of gentamicin and tobramycin. *Ann Intern Med* 1984;*101*:764-9.

16. Hull RD, Raskob GE, Hirsh J, et al. A cost-effectiveness analysis of alternative approaches for long-term treatment of proximal venous thrombosis. *JAMA* 1984;*252*:235-9.

17. Willems JS, Sanders CR, Riddiough MA. Cost-effectiveness of vaccination against pneumococcal pneumonia. *N Engl J Med* 1980;*303*:553-9.

18. Gagnon JP, Osterhaus JT. Proposed drug-drug cost-effectiveness methodology. *Drug Intell Clin Pharm* 1987;*21*:211-6.

19. Rose DN, Schechter CB, Fahs MC, Silver AL. Tuberculosis prevention: cost-effectiveness analysis of isoniazid chemoprophylaxis. *Am J Prev Med* 1988;*4*:102-9.

20. Eisenberg JM, Kitz DS. Savings from outpatient antibiotic therapy for osteomyelitis: economic analysis of a therapeutic strategy. *JAMA* 1986;*255*:1584-8.

21. Zarowitz BJ, Owen H, Popovich J, Pancorbo S. Evaluation of gentamicin premixed admixtures: cost and clinical utility. *Hosp Pharm* 1987;*22*:257-60.

22. Cochran WG. The combination of estimates from different experiments. *Biometrics* 1954; *10*:101-29.

23. Polk RE, Hepler CD. Controversies in antimicrobial therapy: critical analysis of clinical trials. *Am J Hosp Pharm* 1986;*43*:630-40.

24. Besky AS, Sackett DL. When was a "negative" clinical trial big enough? How many patients you needed depends on what you found. *Arch Intern Med* 1985;*145*:709-12.

25. Lipid Research Clinics Program. Coronary primary prevention trial results, II: the relationship of reduction in incidence of coronary heart disease to cholesterol lowering. *JAMA* 1984;*251*:365-74.

26. Hypertension Detection and Follow-Up Program Cooperative Group. Five-year findings of the hypertension detection and follow-up program, I: reduction in mortality in persons with high blood pressure including mild hypertension. *JAMA* 1979;*242*:2562-71.

27. Katz S, ed. The Portugal conference: measuring quality of life and functional status in clinical and epidemiological research. *J Chronic Dis* 1987;*40*:459-650.

28. Briggs GC, Moore BR, Bahado-Singh R, Lange S, Bogh P, Garite TJ. Cost-effectiveness of cefonicid sodium versus cefoxitin sodium for the prevention of postoperative infections after nonelective cesarean section. *Clin Pharm* 1987;*6*:718-21.

29. McGee DL. Probability of developing certain cardiovascular diseases in eight years at specified values of some characteristics. Section 28. In: Kannel WB, Gordon T, eds. The Framingham Study: an epidemiological investigation of cardiovascular disease. U. S. Department of Health, Education, and Welfare Publication (NIH) 74-610. Bethesda, MD: Public Health Service, 1977.

30. Weinstein MC, Stason WB. Cost-effectiveness of interventions to prevent or treat coronary heart disease. *Ann Rev Public Health* 1985;*6*:41-63.

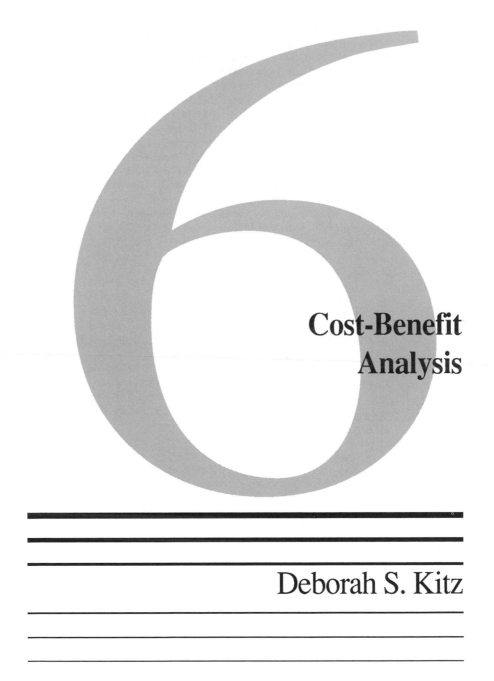

6

Cost-Benefit
Analysis

Deborah S. Kitz

ost-benefit analysis (CBA) is a method for comparing the value of all resources consumed (costs) in providing a program or intervention with the value of the outcome (benefit) from that program or intervention.[1,2] In essence, CBA may be thought of as the "yield" of an "investment." Will the benefits of a program exceed the cost of implementing it? Which program will produce the greatest net benefit?

CBA requires that the costs and benefits both be valued in the same units, usually dollars. If a particular pharmaceutical regimen decreases the need for serum concentration monitoring, the dollar value of the eliminated tests is the benefit. Similarly, if the benefit is lives saved, a dollar value must be assigned to those lives (see Chapter 4 for a discussion of the human capital and willingness-to-pay methods for assigning a monetary value to a life).

Questions Cost-Benefit Analysis Can Answer

Single or multiple interventions may be assessed via CBA. For a single intervention, CBA may be used to determine whether a positive or predetermined minimum return will result from the investment.

Multiple programs with similar or unrelated outcomes may be examined with CBA. Patrick and Woolley, for example, conducted a CBA of three approaches to a pneumococcal pneumonia vaccine program provided by a health maintenance organization (HMO): vaccinating no one, vaccinating all enrollees; or vaccinating all enrollees determined to be at high risk. For each approach, they determined the probability of disease, probability of adverse effects from the vaccine, cost of treating each of these events, and other costs for the HMO and for the patients. The CBA indicated that a program of vaccinating only those patients considered to be at high risk was most appropriate, even when the HMO's costs for identifying high-risk patients were included.[3]

CBA of programs with unrelated outcomes is useful when funds are limited and only one program may be implemented. Should a hospital develop a cephalosporin surveillance program or a cholesterol-lowering program for employees? Which will generate the greatest benefit relative to the cost of implementing each program? Should a city government invest in a prenatal nutrition program, an AIDS awareness program, or three new community health centers?

Steps in Conducting a Cost-Benefit Analysis

The first step in conducting a CBA is to identify clearly the intervention(s), program(s), or therapeutic regimen(s) to be evaluated. Patrick and Woolley included identifying high-risk patients and treating adverse effects from the vaccine as part of the pneumococcal vaccine evaluation. The "program" went beyond administering vaccines and treating disease.[3] For a cephalosporin surveillance program, it is not adequate simply to state that a program will be implemented. Will pharmacists become members of the hospital's infectious disease team? Will all requests for cephalosporins be screened? Will the program be for third-generation cephalosporins only? What are the specific components of the program?

The second step is to identify and value all the resources consumed, or costs of providing each intervention, program, or regimen. Different types of resources should be recognized. In their CBA of an outpatient parenteral antibiotic program, Poretz et al. included expenses for training patients to self-administer drugs, for physician visits, and for supplies.[4]

A hospital pharmacy would include expenses for personnel time (salaries and employee benefits), office space, computer hardware and software, additional telephone lines, and general supplies in a CBA of a cephalosporin surveillance program. A comprehensive comparison of two pharmaceutical therapy regimens would include costs for purchasing each drug, supplies consumed in administering each agent, salary and employee benefit expenses for personnel time (pharmacy and nursing) consumed in preparing and delivering the drug, and hospital resources used to treat untoward effects of each regimen. Shapiro et al. conducted this type of CBA of placebo versus cefazolin prophylaxis in women undergoing vaginal or abdominal hysterectomy and included expenses for hospital days, bacterial cultures, and antimicrobial agents.[5]

Benefits are identified and valued in the third step. Benefits of the cephalosporin surveillance program might include decreased use of third-generation cephalosporins (i.e., lower drug-purchasing budget), and a lower incidence of drug interactions, and associated decreased use of resources to treat untoward events. For the hospital, the value of these benefits is their true cost. For the comparison of two pharmaceutical therapy regimens, the benefits to the hospital of the regimen requiring a shorter duration of treatment would include cost savings from the decreased length of stay.

Recall that if the benefit of an intervention is lives saved, a monetary value must be assigned to those lives. Similarly, if the benefit is fewer days of work missed, actual or estimated patient salary information may be used to assign a dollar value to these days.[4,6]

The fourth step in a CBA is to sum the value of all the costs and of all the benefits of each program, intervention, or regimen. Total costs then may be subtracted from total benefits to determine net benefits (total benefits–total costs = net benefits). Some investigators prefer to compute a cost-to-benefit ratio, while others prefer to calculate a benefit-to-cost ratio. (Although the analytic approach is commonly called cost-benefit analysis, calculating a benefit-to-cost ratio frequently is appropriate because one usually expects benefits to exceed costs, producing a ratio >1:1.)

If the benefit (yield) of an investment in a program (cost) must exceed a minimum dollar value before it is implemented, net benefits should be calculated. A hospital pharmacy may determine that the net benefit of a cephalosporin surveillance program must be at least $50 000 annually. In this case, net benefits should be calculated. Alternatively, a benefit-to-cost ratio should be computed if a criterion for implementing a program is that the benefits must be at least twice as great as the costs (i.e., 2:1 benefit-to-cost ratio), regardless of the absolute value of the benefits and costs. By comparing benefit-to-cost ratios of multiple programs, one can identify the program that produces the greatest "slide for the run," or yield relative to the investment. In some ways, hospital budget allocations to outpatient pharmacy services versus a walk-in clinic versus a trauma program, for example, implicitly compare the "benefit-to-cost ratio" for each program.

Perspective of the Analysis

An important consideration in conducting a CBA and other types of clinical economic evaluations is the perspective of the analysis. For whom are the costs and benefits being assessed? The patient? Departmental manager? Third-party payer? Clinician? Society?

Different resources are considered costs and benefits, and the dollar value of each may vary depending on the perspective from which the analysis is conducted. A hospital pharmacy department would include expenses for a van as part of their costs for an outpatient parenteral therapy program. However, these costs are irrelevant to the patient. Similarly, a patient who is able to return to work considers this a benefit of the outpatient program. This aspect of the program is irrelevant to the pharmacy department, the hospital, and the third-party payer. Patients may incur out-of-pocket expenses for transportation to outpatient follow-up visits. These costs have no impact on the third-party payer, hospital, pharmacy department, or clinician.

Bootman and McGhan also point out that a factor considered to be a benefit from one perspective may be a cost from another perspective.[2] For example, a hospital may view decreased inpatient days as a benefit (under fixed-price payment) of an outpatient parenteral therapy program. However, a patient covered by health insurance that includes a copayment for outpatient care, and 100 percent coverage for inpatient care, would view the decreased inpatient days as a cost. Although insurers would consider the change from inpatient surgical care to outpatient lithotripsy for renal stones a benefit, urologists may consider this to be a cost, particularly if the payment for lithotripter services is lower than for surgical care.

Koplan and Preblud included costs from different perspectives in their clinical economic evaluation of mumps vaccine. For children with mumps, they included estimates of wages lost by parents staying home with the children, expenses for transportation to office visits, cost of the vaccine, and acute care costs.[7] Although they did not place a dollar value on the ability to return to work, Rosenfeldt et al.,[8] and Nevitt et al.[9] did include the ability to return to work as a "benefit" of coronary bypass surgery and of total hip arthroplasty, respectively.

Under fixed-payment schemes for hospital care, the importance of specifying the perspective from which the analysis is being conducted is magnified. These new payment schemes mean that high patient-care expenses generated by the hospital no longer increase third-party payer payments. Extensive and unnecessary use of third-generation cephalosporins, for example, may generate high patient-care costs for the hospital, but do not affect third-party payments. On the other hand, pharmaceutical therapy regimens that shorten the length of stay or eliminate the need for serum concentration monitoring may generate savings for the hospital. From the insurer's perspective, however, no savings will accrue; the payment is fixed. Insurer's costs may increase, however, if a patient receives inpatient care when ambulatory care is feasible and effective.

Fixed-price payment also imposes a relatively new requirement on cost-benefit and other clinical economic analyses performed from the perspective of the hospital: true costs must be assessed. True costs are the value of the resources used in providing a service.[10] Charges, which bear no consistent relationship to costs and often are set to maximize revenue, are irrelevant to assessing hospital expenses or savings under fixed-price payment.

Determining the hospital cost for a service usually is not a trivial task. Determining the cost of different modes of intravenous antibiotic therapy, for example, may involve time and motion studies of personnel time (and assigning salaries and employee benefits) devoted to reconstituting and administering the agent, and hospital expenses for supplies used in each mode.[11] Although determining hospital costs may be a time-consuming, detailed process, it is a critical element of any clinical economic analysis performed from the perspective of the hospital.

Consider the perspective from which the analyses will be conducted in the initial design. More than one perspective may be included in an analysis. However, attention should be devoted to distinguishing the value of costs and value of benefits from each perspective.

Making Assumptions

Frequently, investigators find it necessary to use secondary data sources or to make assumptions about the value of one or more variables in a clinical economic evaluation. This occurs most often when the clinical economic analysis is not being performed in conjunction with the clinical evaluation or when no acceptable retrospective data are available. In the example of the outpatient parenteral therapy program, a hospital may have to estimate annual mileage for a supply-delivery van. Information about the hospital's catchment area and experience of other hospitals may guide the estimates. Nevertheless, the investigator needs to be confident that the value of this variable will not influence the conclusion of the evaluation.

Sensitivity analysis is a method of determining whether the conclusion of an economic evaluation changes when the value of one variable is varied as all other variables are held constant. Will the benefit-to-cost ratio fall below one if expenses for the van mileage are higher than estimated? If personnel expenses for the cephalosporin surveillance program are actually 25 percent higher than estimated, will the net benefits of the program become negative? In other words, sensitivity analysis allows one to determine whether the original conclusions are upheld through the range of variation in the value of the variable in question. Does the benefit-to-cost ratio remain above one through the range of variation (regardless of changes in the value of the ratio)? Do the net benefits remain positive? If the conclusions are upheld, there is a higher degree of validity in the assumption. However, if the conclusions change, efforts should be made to determine the true value of the variable or to state explicitly that the conclusions are "sensitive" to the value of that single variable.

For example, Koplan and Preblud varied the incidence of disease, discount rate (see Chapter 3), and costs per vaccine dose. Under all reasonable ranges of each variable, they found that the benefit-to-cost ratio of mumps vaccine remained above one. Thus, they felt confident of the general finding about the economic aspects of mumps vaccines.[7]

Eisenberg and Kitz included sensitivity analysis in their economic evaluation of outpatient antibiotic therapy for osteomyelitis. Initially, they used information from a previous report indicating that 50 percent of patients could return to their normal routines (e.g., work, school) during outpatient parenteral antibiotic therapy for osteomyelitis. To determine whether the general conclusion was sensitive to the value of this variable, they reanalyzed the data with 0 and 100 percent "return to routine" rates. The original conclusions were upheld under these two values of this variable; benefits would accrue to patients from an outpatient program.[6]

Patrick and Woolley included sensitivity analysis in their CBA of three approaches to pneumococcal pneumonia vaccine for an HMO population. Their overall conclusions about identifying and immunizing high-risk patients did not change when they varied the cost of the vaccine, duration of the program, likelihood of adverse effects, cost of illness, and several other factors.[3]

One approach to sensitivity analysis is to increase and decrease the assumed value of the variable by a significant percent (e.g., 50 or 100 percent). Another approach is to select the mean (e.g., for salaries) for the initial analysis, and then repeat the analysis with the lowest and highest value of the variable.

Cost-Benefit or Cost-Effectiveness Analysis

Cost-benefit and cost-effectiveness analysis are both useful tools for assessing the clinical economic impact of medical care programs or interventions. There are, however, several important distinctions between the two approaches. First, CBA may be applied to single or multiple programs, while cost-effectiveness analysis is applied to multiple programs. Second, CBA may be used to compare programs with disparate outcomes. In contrast, cost-effectiveness analysis is a method for identifying the least costly approach to achieving a single outcome. A third distinction is that CBA requires that all the outcomes or benefits be assigned a dollar value. The outcome or effect is not valued in cost-effectiveness analysis. Some investigators find it distasteful to place a monetary value of a benefit such as lives saved, and thus prefer cost-effectiveness analysis.

Which approach should you use in the clinical pharmacy arena? It depends. A general guideline is that cost-effectiveness analysis is most appropriate when a single effect or outcome can be defined. An effect might be providing antibiotic prophylaxis for patients undergoing surgery for nonperforated appendicitis,[12] or providing postsurgical analgesic therapy. CBA is usually most appropriate when a single program is to be evaluated, or when funds are limited and budget allocation decisions must be made among programs with unrelated outcomes. McGhan et al. point out that CBA is a particularly useful technique for evaluating clinical pharmacy services.[13] Are the costs of implementing a service offset by savings (benefits) from the service? These types of questions will be asked with increasing frequency as hospital administrators and departmental managers respond to cost-containment pressures and incentives created by fixed-price payment.

Cost-Benefit Analysis in the Literature

As noted throughout this section, many of the true CBA in the clinical pharmacy arena have focused on the use of antibiotics. Poretz et al. conducted a CBA of an outpatient parenteral therapy program with ceftriaxone for patients with serious infections. They conducted a telephone survey to determine expenses for training sessions, supplies, physician visits, and transportation to follow-up visits. Income information and days of work missed by patients and a companion was used to assess "productivity" losses. Data also were gathered regarding third-party payer coverage for components of care. The benefit-to-cost ratio of this outpatient therapy program was about 3.7:1; average total weighted benefits were approximately $6600 and costs were about $1800. The authors noted that insurance coverage was less comprehensive for outpatient care than for inpatient care, suggesting that analysis of these types of programs from the patient perspective should consider out-of-pocket expenditures for direct medical care routinely covered when provided as an inpatient.[4]

A type of CBA of another outpatient parenteral therapy program was conducted by Kunkel and Iannini. Their analysis was limited to an estimate of per diem hospital costs (exclusive of ancillary services), a conservative estimate of daily patient wages, and an estimate of nursing time consumed in delivering intravenous antibiotics.[14]

Shapiro et al. incorporated a CBA in a clinical trial of antibiotic prophylaxis for hysterectomy. This approach to conducting an economic evaluation is attractive because data regarding untoward effects, treatment failures, and other clinical parameters are collected concurrently with economic data.[5] A danger of this approach, however, is that particular aspects of therapy, such as serum concentration monitoring, may occur simply because of the clinical trial. Such monitoring would not be part of standard clinical practice, and inadvertently will be included in the economic assessment. It is necessary to exclude from the cost and benefit calculations the clinical trial-related expenses that would not occur in normal practice. Identifying these factors may be difficult, particularly if little information is available about routine practice with a new agent.

The CBA performed by Shapiro et al. included expenses for operative site or urinary tract infections, or febrile morbidity that occurred while the patients were inpatients or within six weeks of discharge following abdominal or vaginal hysterectomy. Although they used charge rather than cost data to assess expenses for hospital days, cultures, and antibiotic agents, the results indicate that the net benefit of prophylaxis versus placebo was about $100 per patient for abdominal hysterectomy and nearly $500 for vaginal hysterectomy.[5]

Vaccination programs also have been evaluated through CBA. In addition to Patrick and Woolley's evaluation of pneumococcal pneumonia vaccines,[3] Koplan and Preblud conducted a CBA of mumps vaccine for children in the U.S.

They included data on disease incidence, vaccine efficacy, mumps encephalitis, hearing loss, and death, and found a benefit-to-cost ratio of at least 7.4:1.[3] Results of other clinical economic evaluations of vaccines have been summarized by Willems and Sanders. They point out that issues regarding target populations for the vaccines, vaccine efficacy, and expenses for administering the vaccines are important and should be examined periodically to reassess the findings of earlier economic evaluations.[15]

Summary

Cost-benefit analysis is an approach to clinical economic assessment. It requires that the costs and benefits both be measured in the same units, usually dollars. A single intervention may be evaluated or multiple interventions with different outcomes may be compared with CBA. Net benefits or a benefit-to-cost ratio may be computed to determine the yield of an "investment" in a diagnostic, therapeutic, or screening intervention.

References

1. Warner KE, Luce BR. Cost-benefit and cost-effectiveness analysis in health care: principles, practice, and potential. Ann Arbor, MI: Health Administration Press, 1982.
2. Bootman JL, McGhan WF. A perspective on the cost-benefit of drug therapy. *Clin Res Pract Drug Reg Aff* 1985;*3*:53-69.
3. Patrick KM, Woolley FR. A cost-benefit analysis of immunization for pneumococcal pneumonia. *JAMA* 1981;*245*:473-7.
4. Poretz DM, Woolard D, Eron LJ, et al. Outpatient use of ceftriaxone: a cost-benefit analysis. *Am J Med* 1984;*10*:77-83.
5. Shapiro M, Schoenbaum SC, Tager IB, Munoz A, Polk BF. Benefit-cost analysis of antimicrobial prophylaxis in abdominal and vaginal hysterectomy. *JAMA* 1983;*249*:1290-4.
6. Eisenberg JM, Kitz DS. Savings from outpatient antibiotic therapy for osteomyelitis: economic analysis of a therapeutic strategy. *JAMA* 1986;*255*:1584-8.
7. Koplan JP, Preblud SR. A benefit-cost analysis of mumps vaccine. *Am J Dis Child* 1982;*136*:362-4.
8. Rosenfeldt FL, Lambert R, Burrows K, Stirling GR. Hospital costs and return to work after coronary bypass surgery. *Med J Aust* 1983;*1*:260-3.
9. Nevitt MC, Epstein WV, Masem M, Murray WR. Work disability before and after total hip arthroplasty: assessment of effectiveness in reducing disability. *Arthritis Rheum* 1984;*27*:410-21.
10. Finkler SA. The distinction between costs and charges. *Ann Intern Med* 1982;*96*:102-9.
11. Eisenberg JM, Koffer H, Finkler SA. Economic analysis of a new drug: potential savings in hospital operating costs from the use of a once-daily regimen of a parenteral cephalosporin. *Rev Infect Dis* 1984;*6*:S909-23.

12. Winslow RE, Dean RE, Harley JW. Acute nonperforating appendicitis: efficacy of brief antibiotic prophylaxis. *Arch Surg* 1983;*118*:651-5.

13. McGhan WF, Rowland CR, Bootman JL. Cost-benefit and cost-effectiveness: methodologies for evaluating innovative pharmaceutical services. *Am J Hosp Pharm* 1978; *35*:133-40.

14. Kunkel MJ, Iannini PB. Cefonicid in a once-daily regimen for treatment of osteomyelitis in an ambulatory setting. *Rev Infect Dis* 1984;*6*:S865-9.

15. Willems JS, Sanders CR. Cost-effectiveness and cost-benefit analyses of vaccines. *J Infect Dis* 1982;*144*:486-93.

7

Decision Analysis and Pharmacoeconomic Evaluations

Judith T. Barr
Gerald E. Schumacher

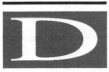ecisions are a fact of everyday life. Whether at home or in clinical practice, decisions always must be made. From a decision as mundane as whether to go to a movie or a concert to a clinical consideration of which antibiotic to select, decisions span a range of complexity. Using the techniques of reasoned guess, gut-reaction, or intuition in our decision-making process, our usual course of action is to implicitly consider the decision, its options, and possibly the near-term consequences. If other considerations are recognized, they somehow are factored into the process in an ad hoc juggling act. This chapter demonstrates that the decision process can be improved and that decision analysis can be an important tool in pharmacoeconomic evaluations.

Our intuitive decision-making capabilities are limited, and we rarely attempt an explicit examination of all factors affecting the decision and its outcome. But our decisions can be improved through the use of the explicit structure and quantitative techniques of decision analysis—a systematic approach to decision-making under uncertain conditions. Since few decisions are accompanied with absolute certainty of the consequences of their outcomes, decision analysis can be used to assist the decision maker to identify the available options, predict the consequences or outcomes of each option, assess the likelihood or probability of the identified possible outcomes, determine the value of each outcome, and select the decision option that will provide the best pay-off. Decision analysis not only forces an explicit, orderly, and careful consideration of a variety of important issues, but it also provides insight into the process of decision making.

Decision analysis is explicit—it forces one to structure the decision as well as identify the consequences of the possible outcomes. It is quantitative—it forces one to assign numbers to probability estimates and outcome valuations. It is prescriptive—the analysis identifies the decision route to take to maximize the expected value of the decision.

The origins of decision analysis, as well as many of the techniques presented in this book, can be traced to the British during World War II when principles of game theory, systems analysis, and operations research were applied to decisions involving the allocation of scarce resources. By the 1950s, these techniques were combined in the business world into the evolving field of decision analysis. The late 1950s saw the beginning of medical applications[1] and the approach reached the medical literature in the early and mid-1970s.[2-4] Cost-benefit, cost-effectiveness, and cost-utility are extensions of decision analytic technology.[5]

Decision analysis is now an integral component of business school curricula as universities prepare future managers to make better allocative and strategic decisions. From Raiffa's classic lectures[6] to decision-support computer packages, decision analysis is now central to business, economic, and health decisions.

In healthcare fields, a recent review article identified nearly 200 decision analytic citations from the clinical literature that assist in decisions related to 1 or more of 13 categories of clinical problems.[5] In the medical community, decision analysis is being "institutionalized." The Society for Medical Decision Making was established in 1977 and publishes a quarterly journal, *Medical Decision Making*; clinical decision consultation services have been established to provide assistance with complex patient-specific decisions;[7] and the American Association of Medical Colleges recommended the inclusion of clinical decision analysis in the undergraduate medical curriculum.

This chapter provides the opportunity to apply decision analysis to the process of combining pharmacoeconomic considerations of the business world with the associated health consequences in clinical settings. The steps and techniques of the decision-analytic process are illustrated by their application to a decision facing a pharmacy and therapeutics (P&T) committee.

Decision analysis is a method with techniques to analyze situations. But perhaps more importantly, the use of decision analysis engenders an attitude towards the problem or decision: to think more analytically; to force the consideration of consequences of actions; to explicitly recognize that uncertainty is present, to estimate the degree of uncertainty, and to assess the attitude towards risk; to determine which are the relevant outcome measures; and to value the preferences for the alternative outcomes.

The Case

Consider that alphazorin and omegazorin are the only FDA-approved members of a new (fictional) class of antibiotic. Both are effective against gram-negative bacteria that are resistant to multiple antibiotics, and both block the transfer

Table 1. Comparison of Alphazorin and Omegazorin Characteristics

	Alphazorin	Omegazorin
Cost of ten-day course of therapy	$1100	$700
Frequency of dosage regimen	q8h	q6h
Resistance rate	5%	12%
Drug-related toxicities		
gastrointestinal toxicity	7%	10%
hepatotoxicity	1.5%	3.5%
hematotoxicity	0.4%	1.5%
Subtherapeutic response rate	10%	15%
Characteristics of serum drug concentration at toxic/nontoxic cut-off level		
predictive value positive	80%	90%
predictive value negative	90%	85%
Characteristics of serum drug concentration at subtherapeutic/resistant cut-off level		
predictive value positive	90%	87.5%
predictive value negative	80%	90%

of extrachromosomal resistance factors between bacterial cells. In clinical trials, 95 percent of the cases of gram-negative septicemia were susceptible to alphazorin; 87 percent were susceptible to omegazorin. Although omegazorin has a higher incidence of drug-associated toxicity, both must be maintained within a narrow therapeutic range. Toxic adverse effects for both include diarrhea and vomiting (gastrointestinal toxicity), hepatic enzyme alterations (hepatotoxicity), and megakarocyte suppression (hematotoxicity).

The initial expenses of a ten-day course of intravenous alphazorin q8h are $1100 for the direct and indirect costs associated with drug acquisition and storage and $240 for dispensing and administration; for omegazorin q6h, the costs are $700 and $320, respectively. While alphazorin has the higher costs, it also has the higher percentage of successfully treated gram-negative bacteremia and a lower incidence of drug-associated toxicity. Important characteristics for each antibiotic are summarized in Table 1.

The P&T committee has decided to approve the addition of at least one of these antibiotics to the formulary, but which one? How can the committee combine all the factors necessary to reach its decision: the cost of the antibiotics, the difference in susceptibility/resistance rates, the varying toxicity and subtherapeutic response rates, and the classification accuracy of the serum drug concentrations?

The application of decision analysis involves five major steps:

1. Identify the decision, including the selection of the decision options to be studied. Bound the timeframe of the decision.
2. Structure the decision and the consequences of each option over time.

3. Assess the probability that each consequence will occur.
4. Determine the value of each outcome (e.g., in dollars, quality-adjusted life years saved, utilities).
5. Select the option with the highest expected value.

Applying the steps and structure of decision analysis, we will evaluate the alphazorin and omegazorin case. The definitions and conventions of clinical decision analysis as presented by Weinstein and Fineberg are used throughout the chapter.[8]

Identify and Bound the Decision

The ground rules of the decision are set at this stage. Who will be the decision maker? Whose perspectives will be considered? What is the decision and what options will be considered? Over what time span will the consequences be analyzed? The answers to these questions are necessary to properly structure the decision and to collect the appropriate data.

WHO WILL BE THE DECISION MAKER?

This question is asked primarily to determine from what perspective the analysis is to be conducted. Is it from the point of view of the pharmacy department, the hospital, an insurance company, or a health maintenance organization? If the decision's impact on the financial resources of a unit is being considered, the type of unit will make a difference as to whether to measure costs or charges, which costs or charges to include, and over what time period they should be collected. For example, if the decision is being considered based on the financial impact to the pharmacy department, only the drug acquisition costs and the pharmacy-associated direct and indirect costs of the drug's storage, dispensing, administration, and monitoring would be included. On the other hand, a health maintenance organization would consider all inpatient and outpatient charges and costs related to the entire episode of care; an insurance company would be interested in the episodes of care charges covered under the terms of the insurance policy.

In this case, the analysis will be conducted from the hospital's perspective. Therefore, in addition to the drug-related costs, the costs of all hospital goods and services during the hospitalization period generally are included in the study. However, since the P&T committee already has decided to add at least one of the drugs to the formulary, it is unnecessary to calculate the nondrug-related costs of an uncomplicated, ten-day hospital stay for intravenous treatment of similar gram-negative infections, because they are the same for both alphazorin and omegazorin. Rather, the additional direct and indirect costs associated with the drugs and the consequences of their respective therapies will be included: drug acquisition, storage, and dispensing; drug administration; and additional monitoring and laboratory costs, hospital stay, and pharmacokinetic and infectious disease consultations due to bacterial resistance, adverse toxic or subtherapeutic consequences of the antibiotic, or of misclassification errors of the serum drug concentrations.

WHAT IS THE DECISION, ITS OPTIONS, AND THE DECISION CRITERION?

The P&T committee has decided to add at least one member of the new antibiotic class to its formulary and also to add both if the additional cost of the drug and drug-related therapy with the second antibiotic is no more than 15 percent higher than the less expensive one. Therefore, the first decision is "Which of the two antibiotics definitely will be added to the formulary?" This is the decision for which the decision tree will be constructed and the analysis performed. The decision options are alphazorin and omegazorin.

What decision criterion is to be used to select between the two antibiotics? The criterion is linked to what type of analysis is being performed. If cost and lives saved are selected, it would be a cost-effectiveness study; if cost and utilities are measured, it is a cost-utility assessment. All of the previously described pharmacoeconomic analyses can use the steps and structure of clinical decision analysis; only the unit of outcome measurement (decision criterion) would differ.

The committee decided to limit its decision to the expected cost of treating an infection or a cost minimization study.[9] To standardize the analysis, it selected gram-negative septicemia as the base case, since it is representative of the type of infections to be treated with these antibiotics. Now that the decision criterion is clarified, the decision maker must select the antibiotic that results in the lower expected cost for treatment of this representative infection.

In the "scientific notation" of decision analysis, a choice node (a square) indicates a point in time when the decision maker can select one of several options or actions. This choice node is placed at the far left and designates the beginning of the decision tree; the possible options (alphazorin and omegazorin) then originate as branches to the right of this initial node. This tree provides an explicit structure for this cost study. The start of the decision tree is shown in Figure 1.

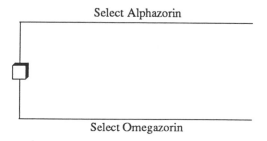

Figure 1. Initial choice node of decision tree to select addition to formulary.

Following the decision criterion, the branch option with the lower expected cost will be the antibiotic selected for addition to the formulary. If the expected cost of the other branch is no more than 15 percent higher than the preferred option, that antibiotic also will be included.

OVER WHAT TIME SPAN WILL THE ANALYSIS APPLY?

The time period will begin with the initiation of either antibiotic to treat gram-negative septicemia (analysis limited to culture-confirmed cases) and end with the discontinuation of antibiotic therapy for septicemia or termination of treatment for drug-induced toxicity.

Develop a Decision Tree—Structure the Decision and Its Consequences Over Time

This is one of the most powerful features of decision analysis. Forcing the decision maker to explicitly structure the situation changes the intuitive process into one in which the thought process is clearly articulated. Laying out the tree prods the decision maker into identifying the relationships that exist between the decision options and possible future consequences. The tree becomes a tool to assist in thinking through a decision as well as to assist in communications among individuals and departments working on the same analysis. With a decision tree, coworkers can identify where they agree or disagree in the considered alternatives and consequences, suggest additional consequences that must be "bushed out," or recommend that a branch be trimmed.

Given the decision options originating from the initial choice node, the consequences of each action must be determined. These consequences are chronologically structured over time in a decision tree by asking a series of "what if" questions. This section structures the decision tree and details the consequences of the actions. The next section examines how likely each of these consequences is to occur; and the section after that determines the cost implications of each option.

What if septicemic patients are given alphazorin? Follow the alphazorin branch of the decision tree in Figure 2 as the consequences are described. The omegazorin portion of the tree is displayed in Figure 3. For the moment, focus only on the tree structures—their branches and nodes. The dollar values in the bubbles, the numbers near the chance nodes, the path number, and the cost column are explained in following sections.

First, the outcome at this branch is no longer under the control of the decision maker; some of the patients will respond, and some of them will not. A chance node (indicated by a circle inserted in the appropriate branch) notes the point in time when the decision maker loses control of the decision process, when future events are beyond the control of the decision maker and the outcome is uncertain.

In this case, the chance node is inserted in the alphazorin branch, and the response possibilities originate from this node.

If the fever recedes and the laboratory results indicate response to the antibiotic (the response branch), patients may continue uneventfully for the balance of the ten-day course of therapy, or they may develop three principal types of toxic reactions: (1) gastrointestinal (GI) effects such as nausea, vomiting, and

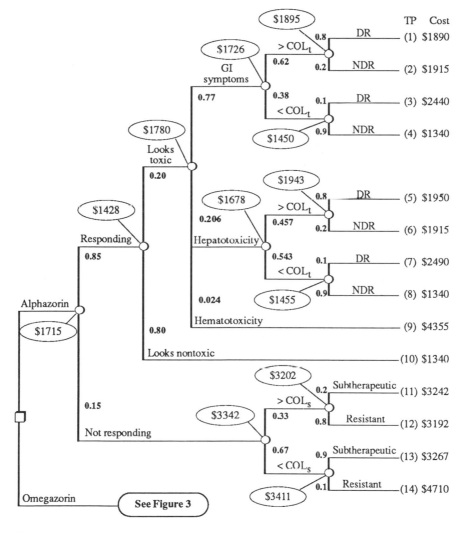

Figure 2. Alphazorin portion of structured decision tree including probabilities, outcome valuations in dollars, and expected cost of the alphazorin option. COL_s = subtherapeutic cut-off level; COL_t = toxic cut-off level; DR = drug-related; GI = gastrointestinal; NDR = nondrug-related; TP = tree path.

diarrhea, which usually occur on day 3 of therapy; (2) hepatotoxicity with elevated enzymes and reduced liver failure (usually occur on day 5); and (3) hematotoxicity (usually occur on day 6).

However, not all toxic symptoms in these patients are related to alphazorin; rather, they can be associated with other medications or the nature of the underlying illness. To determine if the toxicity is or is not drug-related, serum alpha-

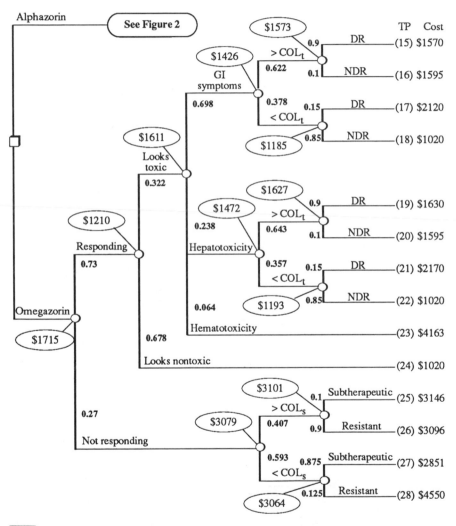

Figure 3. Omegazorin portion of structured decision tree including probabilities, outcome valuations in dollars, and expected cost of the omegazorin option. COL$_s$ = subtherapeutic cut-off level; COL$_t$ = toxic cut-off level; DR = drug-related; GI = gastrointestinal; NDR = nondrug-related; TP = tree path.

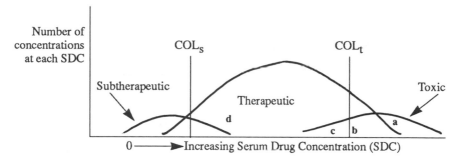

Figure 4. Frequency of subtherapeutic, therapeutic, and toxic patients at increasing serum drug concentrations. COL_s = subtherapeutic cut-off levels; COL_t = toxic cut-off levels

zorin levels (SAL) are used. Therefore, a chance node with two branches follows each of the indicated toxicities—either the concentration is above or below the toxic cut-off level (COL_t).

It is rare when a test clearly separates one patient population from another; generally, there are areas of overlap.[10] As shown in Figure 4, most patients above the COL_t have drug-related toxicity ("a" in Figure 4), but some with nondrug-related symptoms also have high levels ("b"). The majority of patients with concentrations below the COL_t do not have drug-associated symptoms ("d"), but there are some patients with alphazorin-related toxicities who have levels below COL_t ("c"). Therefore, to display both the correct and incorrect classifications based on COL_t, a chance node with drug- and nondrug-related branches follow all >COL_t and <COL_t results.

Additional consequences occur at many of these branches; for example, the misclassification of a concentration below the COL_t as nondrug-related, when the symptoms really were associated with drug toxicity, can lead to continuation of the antibiotic, the development of more serious adverse effects, and longer hospital stays. To simplify the decision tree, such additional consequences are not further detailed as additional branches, but are considered explicitly in the cost implication section.

In the "not responding" branch, serum drug concentrations are ordered to distinguish between two patient populations: (1) those with bacterial infections susceptible to alphazorin, but receiving dosages that are achieving subtherapeutic concentrations; and (2) those with bacterial infections that are resistant to the drug. Again, the SAL is used to differentiate between the two populations, but misclassification errors occur when the subtherapeutic/therapeutic cut-off level (COL_s) is applied. Most concentrations above COL_s are from nonresponding patients with resistant organisms; however, some are from patients with subtherapeutic responses who will be switched unnecessarily to another antibiotic when a dosage adjustment is all that is needed. On the other branch, the majority of patients with concentrations below COL_s have susceptible infections and need their dosage increased. But patients with low levels and resistant organisms are placed at risk because, rather than switching them to a more appropriate antibiotic, the alphazorin dosage is increased in response to the low SAL, and a course of ineffective therapy is lengthened.

The alphazorin section of the decision tree, complete with all decision options and drug selection consequences chronologically arranged from left to right, is complete. All decisions under the control of the decision maker are indicated by choice nodes; all outcomes left to chance and beyond the control of the decision maker are indicated by chance nodes. There are 14 possible outcomes in this section, each indicated by a number on the right side of a path in Figure 2. A path is a sequence of action and events beginning with the decision at the initial choice node and following the consequences of that decision in a unique line from left to right through subsequent chance and/or choice nodes.

The omegazorin section of the decision tree is displayed in Figure 3. The consequences of selecting omegazorin are represented by the same structure as the alphazorin option. If the consequences are the same, why are not the two antibiotics considered equal? First, the likelihood or probability of occurrence of each of the consequences differs between the two drugs, and second, the cost of the antibiotics as well as the cost of each decision path differ. These are examined in the following two sections.

Assess Probabilities

The probabilities associated with the various consequences for each antibiotic have been calculated from a large randomized study of patients with possible gram-negative septicemia: half of them received alphazorin and the other half, omegazorin. The first 1000 patients receiving alphazorin and having gram-negative bacteremia confirmed by culture provide the alphazorin probability data set. The same method was used for the omegazorin probability estimates. The P&T committee has determined that the patient conditions and consequences in the clinical trial are representative of the patients at this hospital. The outcome results of the 2000 patients are summarized in Table 2.

The sum of the probabilities of all consequences originating from a chance node must be 1.0; therefore, it is essential that all possible consequences be identified at each chance node. Because there is a 100 percent certainty that something will happen at each chance node, nodes with probabilities totaling less than 1.0 do not have all consequences identified and, thus, have been incompletely specified. The probabilities associated with each branch originating from a chance node are displayed adjacent to the respective branch. They have been calculated as follows.

Of the 1000 patients receiving alphazorin, 850 (85 percent) responded with temperature reduction and change in the blood picture; 150 (15 percent) did not

Table 2. Frequency of Outcome for 1000 Patients Receiving Alphazorin and 1000 Patients Receiving Omegazorin*

Drug and Outcome						Decision Path
Alphazorin, responding					850	
Symptoms resembling toxicity				170		
Gastrointestinal toxicity			131			
> COL_t		81				
drug-related	65					(1)
not drug-related	16					(2)
< COL_t		50				
drug-related	5					(3)
not drug-related	45					(4)
Hepatotoxicity			35			
> COL_t		16				
drug-related	13					(5)
not drug-related	3					(6)
< COL_t		19				
drug-related	2					(7)
not drug-related	17					(8)
Hematotoxicity			4			(9)
No toxic symptoms				680		(10)
Alphazorin, not responding					150	
> COL_s				50		
subtherapeutic			10			(11)
resistant			40			(12)
< COL_s				100		
subtherapeutic			90			(13)
resistant			10			(14)
Omegazorin, responding					730	
Symptoms resembling toxicity				235		
Gastrointestinal toxicity			164			
> COL_t		102				
drug-related	91					(15)
not drug-related	11					(16)
< COL_t		62				
drug-related	11					(17)
not drug-related	51					(18)
Hepatotoxicity			56			
> COL_t		36				
drug-related	32					(19)
not drug-related	4					(20)
< COL_t		20				
drug-related	3					(21)
not drug-related	17					(22)
Hematotoxicity			15			(23)
No toxic symptoms				495		(24)
Omegazorin, not responding					270	
> COL_s				110		
subtherapeutic			10			(25)
resistant			100			(26)
< COL_s				160		
subtherapeutic			140			(27)
resistant			20			(28)

COL_s = subtherapeutic cut-off level; COL_t = toxic cut-off level.

respond. The probabilities of response/nonresponse are entered in the decision tree on the two branches originating from the alphazorin branch at the initial choice node. Of the 850 responding patients, 680 (80 percent) had no toxic symptoms and 170 (20 percent) did have possible drug-related toxicities. Of the 170 patients with toxic symptoms, 131 (77 percent) had gastrointestinal toxicity, 35 (20.6 percent) had elevated liver function enzymes suggesting drug-related hepatotoxicity, and 4 (2.4 percent) had a marked reduction in platelet numbers and function.

Serum alphazorin concentrations were determined on all patients with toxic symptoms. Eighty-one of 131 (62 percent) GI symptoms were associated with concentrations above COL_t. The results for hepatoxicity and hematotoxicity are 16 of 35 (45.7 percent) and 4 of 4 (100 percent), respectively. But, as discussed earlier, the toxic cut-off level cannot cleanly separate the drug-related from the nondrug-related population.

Measures of a test's predictive ability, predictive value positive (PV^+), and predictive value negative (PV^-) can be helpful. (See Table 1 for predictive value information for both alphazorin and omegazorin.) Predictive value positive answers the question: Given a concentration above the toxic cut-off, what is the probability that the concentration is from a patient who has drug-related toxicity? For SAL, the PV^+ is 80 percent. Conversely, the probability that a level above COL_t is from a patient whose toxicity is not drug-related is represented by the mathematical expression $(1-PV^+)$, or 20 percent for alphazorin. Similarly, the predictive value negative answers the question: Given a concentration below the toxic cut-off, what is the probability that the concentration is from a patient who does not have drug-related toxicity? For SAL, the PV^- is 90 percent. The probability that a concentration below COL_t is from a drug-related toxic patient is $(1-PV^-)$ or 10 percent.

In the nonresponding population, 100 of 150 patients (67 percent) had concentrations below the subtherapeutic cut-off level; 50 of 150 (33 percent) were above COL_s. At this lower cut-off level, the predictive value positive is the proportion of levels below COL_s that are from subtherapeutic patients or 90 percent for alphazorin. Ten percent of concentrations below COL_s are associated with resistant organisms. PV^- is the proportion of levels above COL_s that are from nonsubtherapeutic patients (those with resistant organisms) or 80 percent for alphazorin. The remaining 20 percent are associated with patients whose concentrations are above COL_s, but who need a higher dosage to obtain a therapeutic response.

Different probabilities are associated with the population receiving omegazorin. Fewer of the causative organisms were susceptible to this drug (88 vs. 95 percent), and there was a higher incidence of drug-related toxicity (15.0 vs. 8.9 percent). Of the 1000 patients receiving this medication, 730 (73 percent) responded to the medication; 495 of these (67.8 percent) had no toxic symptoms, and 235 (32.2 percent) did. Of the patients with possible toxicity, 164 (69.8 percent) had GI signs, 56 (23.8 percent) had elevated liver function enzymes, and 15 (6.4 percent) had marked platelet dysfunction.

At omegazorin's COL_t, 90 percent of the concentrations above COL_t are from patients with drug-related toxicities ($PV^+ = 0.90$); 85 percent below COL_t are from patients whose symptoms are not associated with omegazorin toxicity ($PV^- = 0.85$). At COL_s, 87.5 percent of concentrations below COL_s are from patients with a subtherapeutic dosage. Ninety percent of the levels above COL_s are associated with resistant organisms.

It must be noted that this is an ideal database, one rarely found in the clinical literature. As more clinical decisions are based on cost as well as efficacy, it is essential that the collection of this type of probabilistic patient outcome information becomes routine practice and a component of clinical trials. An accurate cost-impact assessment is not possible unless it is linked to the probabilities of clinical consequences. Until these data are available, probability estimates can be generated using expert opinions, Delphi techniques, and meta-analysis of literature reports. The reader is referred to other sources for a critique of probability estimates resulting from methods other than direct clinical studies.[11,12]

Value Outcomes

The P&T committee has decided to value the outcomes by determining the monetary value of drug, drug-related, and drug-induced costs per septicemic case. The drug costs include the direct and indirect expenses of drug acquisition and storage: a ten-day course is $1100 for alphazorin and $700 for omegazorin. Drug-related costs consist of an $8 direct and indirect cost each time either drug is administered. Alphazorin is administered q8h, resulting in a cost of $240 for ten days of therapy; omegazorin is q6h, costing $320 for the same length of drug administration. When a change of therapy is indicated due to suspected bacterial resistance, a ten-day course of intravenous betasporin is initiated, costing $1200 in drug and $240 in drug-related costs. For a more thorough review of cost determination and analysis, see Chapter 3.

Drug-induced costs are those incurred due to the follow-up created by less than optimal response to either alphazorin or omegazorin. These costs, calculated by the input component method and incorporating direct and indirect expenses, include $450/extra day of hospital stay, additional laboratory tests ($25/drug concentration, $20/liver function studies, $15/platelet count), component therapy ($150/packed red cell transfusion and platelet concentrate), $50/pharmacokinetic consult, and $200/infectious disease and hematology consults (charges).

The inputs and associated costs required for each path in the alphazorin section of the decision tree are summarized in Table 3 and for omegazorin in Table 4. The path costs are entered at the right of each path on the decision tree sections in Figures 2 and 3.

Table 3. Outcome Costs Associated with Consequences of Alphazorin-Treated Septicemia

Path	Clinical Condition	Drug	Drug-Related	Drug-Induced a*	b†	c‡	d**	e††	Total
1	Alpha-related GI symptoms, > COL_t, drug adjusted	$1100	$240	$450	$50	$	$50	$	$1890
2	Non-alpha-related GI symptoms, > COL_t, drug reduced unnecessarily	1100	240	450	75		50		1915
3	Alpha-related GI symptoms, < COL_t, delay in drug adjustment	1100	240	900	100		100		2440
4	Non-alpha-related GI symptoms, < COL_t, drug therapy continued	1100	240						1340
5	Alpha-related liver toxicity, > COL_t, drug adjusted	1100	240	450	50	60	50		1950
6	Non-alpha-related liver toxicity, > COL_t, drug reduced unnecessarily	1100	240	450	75		50		1915
7	Alpha-related liver toxicity, < COL_t, delay in drug adjustment	1100	240	900	50	100	100		2490
8	Non-alpha-related liver toxicity, < COL_t, drug therapy continued	1100	240						1340
9	Alpha-related hematotoxicity, drug switched (6 d alpha, 4 d beta)	1140	240	1800		675	100	400	4355
10	Uncomplicated response	1100	240						1340
11	Subtherapeutic response, > COL_s, alpha 3 d, changed to beta 10 d	1530	312	1350			50		3242
12	Resistant, > COL_s, alpha 3 d; switch to beta 10 d	1530	312	1350					3192
13	Subtherapeutic response, < COL_s, alpha adjusted 13 d	1430	312	1350	75		100		3267
14	Resistant, < COL_s, adjust alpha (5 d); then switch to beta 10 d	1750	360	2250	50		100	200	4710

*Extra hospital day at $450/d.
†Drug concentration at $25/level.
‡Extra laboratory costs including component therapy.
**Pharmacokinetic consultation at $50.
††Hematology or infectious disease consultation at $200.
COL_s = subtherapeutic cut-off level; COL_t = toxic cut-off level; GI = gastrointestinal.

Table 4. Outcome Costs Associated with Consequences of Omegazorin-Treated Septicemia

Path	Clinical Condition	Drug	Drug-Related	Drug-Induced					Total
				a*	b†	c‡	d**	e††	
15	Omega-related GI symptoms, > COL_t, drug adjusted	$700	$320	$450	$50	$	$50	$	$1570
16	Non-omega-related GI symptoms, > COL_t, drug reduced unnecessarily	700	320	450	75		50		1595
17	Omega-related GI symptoms, < COL_t, delay in drug adjustment	700	320	900	100		100		2120
18	Non-omega-related GI symptoms, < COL_t, drug therapy continued	700	320						1020
19	Omega-related liver toxicity, > COL_t, drug adjusted	700	320	450	50	60	50		1630
20	Non-omega-related liver toxicity, > COL_t, drug reduced unnecessarily	700	320	450	75		50		1595
21	Omega-related liver toxicity, < COL_t, delay in drug adjustment	700	320	900	50	100	100		2170
22	Non-omega-related liver toxicity, < COL_t, drug therapy continued	700	320						1020
23	Omega-related hematotoxicity, drug switched (6 d alpha, 4 d beta)	900	288	1800		675	100	400	4163
24	Uncomplicated response	700	320						1020
25	Subtherapeutic response, > COL_s, omega 3 d, changed to beta 10 d	1410	336	1350			50		3146
26	Resistant, > COL_s, omega 3 d; switch to beta 10 d	1410	336	1350					3096
27	Subtherapeutic response, < COL_s, omega adjusted 13 d	910	416	1350	75		100		2851
28	Resistant, < COL_s, adjust omega (5 d); then switch to beta 10 d	1550	400	2250	50		100	200	4550

*Extra hospital day at $450/d.
†Drug concentration at $25/level.
‡Extra laboratory costs including component therapy.
**Pharmacokinetic consultation at $50.
††Hematology or infectious disease consultation at $200.
COL_s = subtherapeutic cut-off level; COL_t = toxic cut-off level; GI = gastrointestinal.

Choose the Preferred Course of Action—Calculate the Expected Cost for Each Decision Outcome

How does one combine the various decision options, probability estimates, and outcome valuations to choose the preferred course of action? How does one "solve" a decision tree?

First, it is necessary to break the decision tree into its component parts and analyze smaller sections. This is done in reverse order of the tree's development by starting from the right and working back to the initial decision or choice node on the left. The process is called averaging out and folding back, since each path's outcome value is weighted by its probability of occurrence (averaging out) and working from right to left, from outcomes to options (folding back).

At each chance node, outcome values (costs) are combined with, and weighted by, their respective probability of occurring. This yields an expected cost at each chance node. For illustration, a section of the alphazorin portion of the decision tree is reproduced in Figure 5. Starting on the right with those patients who have GI symptoms and have serum concentrations above the COL_t, 80 percent will have alphazorin-related toxicity with an associated average cost of treatment of $1890. However, 20 percent of the patients with high serum concentrtions will not have drug-related toxicity; their dosage will be reduced unnecessarily and will result in an average cost of $1915 for this path. To calculate the expected cost of patients with alphazorin concentrations above COL_t, the cost of each outcome is weighted by the probability of its occurrence and then added to the weighted costs of all other outcomes originating from the same chance node.

$$(80\%) (\$1890) + (20\%) (\$1915) = \$1895 \qquad \text{Eq. 1}$$

For patients with concentrations below COL_t, 90 percent of the symptoms will be nondrug-related at a cost of $1340. However, 10 percent of these concentrations will be from patients with drug-related toxicity. Their dosage will be continued, leading to additional toxicity and extended hospitalizations at an av-

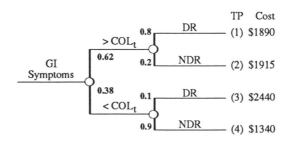

Figure 5. Section of alphazorin portion of decision tree. COL_t = toxic cut-off level; DR = drug-related; GI = gastrointestinal; NDR = nondrug-related; TP = tree path.

erage cost of $2440. The expected costs of patients with GI symptoms whose concentrations are below COL_t are:

$$(90\%) (\$1340) + (10\%) (\$2440) = \$1450 \qquad \text{Eq. 2}$$

The next step back to the origin or left of the tree requires the determination of the expected cost of all patients with GI symptoms. At the next chance node, the expected costs of patients with drug concentrations above and below COL_t are combined with their respective probability of occurring. There is a 62 percent probability that the concentration will be above COL_t; that condition has an expected cost of $1895. There also is a probability of 38 percent that the concentration will be below COL_t with an expected cost of $1450. Therefore, the average expected cost of all patients with GI symptoms is:

$$(62\%) (\$1895) + (38\%) (\$1450) = \$1726 \qquad \text{Eq. 3}$$

The expected cost has been calculated for each chance node and appears in the bubble attached to each node. The averaging out and folding back process continues until the expected costs are determined for the two branches originating from the initial choice node. These have been calculated and appear in Figures 2 and 3; the expected cost of the alphazorin option is $1715 and of the omegazorin branch, $1715.

Thus, although omegazorin's acquisition price is $400 lower than alphazorin, the institutional costs associated with omegazorin's higher resistance rate and increased drug-related toxicities increase the total septicemia treatment costs to the same as that for alphazorin. Previously, the P&T committee may have selected only omegazorin based on the $400 cost differential, but clinical decision analysis provided the framework within which they were able to identify and value the consequences. If this decision analysis had been extended to include utility assessments as well as costs for each of the outcome paths, it is likely that a cost-utility analysis would favor the more expensive alphazorin due to the higher incidence of negative outcomes with omegazorin.

From the identification of the decision options, the time frame, the decision criteria, and the objectives of the decision maker; through the structuring of the decision and the identification of all consequences; to probability assessment and outcome valuation; the decision now has had an explicit, structured, analytic, and quantitative assessment with a preferred action course identified—both antibiotics will be added to the department's formulary.

Literature Examples of Analytic Studies in Therapeutic Decisions

In addition to selected examples of cost-effectiveness and cost-utility studies using an underlying decision tree structure,[13-23] three published case studies apply decision analysis to therapeutic selection and/or action.[24-26] All three appeared in the "Clinical Decision Making Rounds at the New England Medical Center," a case prepared by that service for selected issues of the quarterly journal, *Medical Decision Making*. These articles are valuable examples of therapeutic applications of clinical decision analysis and also describe the sources and quality of data used in the analytic process.

Gottlieb and Pauker described a patient with acute myelogenous leukemia who now likely has *Candida* esophagitis and, quite possibly, disseminated fungal infection. But without a confirmation of systemic mycosis, do the known risks of systemic amphotericin therapy outweigh the possible benefits? A tree was constructed, probabilities estimated from the literature and then modified by expert opinion, and the outcome of each action consequence measured as quality-adjusted months, a metric to combine quality and quantity of life. Based on this analysis and the assessment that the patient had at least a 30 percent probability of systemic mycosis, the amphotericin action option was estimated to yield the highest quality-adjusted life months.[24]

Plante and Pauker used a computer program, Decision Maker, to construct a decision tree with 773 (!) paths to decide if a patient with enterococcal endocarditis and a possible history of penicillin hypersensitivity should receive penicillin. Probabilities were determined from the literature and outcomes valued using a complex morbidity and mortality utility scale. The article has an extensive discussion of data sources and quality. Analysis indicated penicillin as the preferred course of therapy based on the patient's clinical condition and other data sources.[25]

Cuchural et al. examined whether immunosuppression should or should not be continued in a transplant patient with malignant melanoma. Probabilities were estimated from the literature and the outcome was expressed in quality-adjusted life expectancy. This outcome unit used the patient's preferences to determine the quality adjustment for the various outcome states. Based on the patient's preferences, his past history, and the probabilities from the literature, the decrease in life expectancy associated with an additional melanoma did not warrant the discontinuance of the immunosuppressive drugs.[26]

Two additional articles applied decision analytic methodology to the interpretation of therapeutic drug monitoring concentrations. Eraker and Sasse conducted a Bayesian assessment of digoxin concentrations;[27] Schumacher and Barr constructed a decision tree to guide the therapeutic response to theophylline concentrations.[28] Both provide additional insight into the applications and methods of decision analysis, and discuss the additional information that can be gained from the use of this process.

Since the application of decision analysis to clinical situations is relatively new, it is important to critically examine the assumptions, the specification of the model, and the generalizability of the conclusions of published reports. This is illustrated by two recent articles that apply decision analysis to the question of whether antibiotic prophylaxis is cost-effective for travelers' diarrhea[29] and for dental procedures in patients with artificial joints.[30]

Both studies used a decision tree to organize the analysis and identify the consequences of the decision options. In the dental prophylaxis study, probability assessments were derived from literature studies; the travelers' diarrhea investigators, citing conflicting and incomplete published reports, obtained probability estimates from six experts in infectious disease epidemiology, diarrheal disease treatment and prophylaxis, and pharmacology. The dental prophylaxis group measured their outcomes in both dollars as well as quality-adjusted life-year (QALY) saved; in the notation of this book, it is more correctly titled a cost-utility study with cost per QALY saved as the unit of the measurement. However, in the travelers' diarrhea study, only the costs of the drug, drug reactions, incapacitation days, hospital days, and chronic diarrhea were included; there was no measure of effect. Both reports included sensitivity analyses that examine the effect of changes of probabilities and costs on the conclusions.

Decision Analytic Computer Support

Decision support systems provide the computational power to conduct complex analyses with multiple branches and a range of probabilities and outcome assessments. Several were originally developed for medical application, such as: D-Maker (Digital Medicine, 39 South Main Street, Hanover, NH 03755) and SMLTREE: The All Purpose Decision Tree Builder (Jim Hollenberg, 445 East 68th Street, Apartment 11-P, New York, NY 10021). Others were designed for a generic audience and can be adapted for clinical applications, such as: Arborist: Decision Tree Software (Texas Instruments, Dallas, TX 78769) and Supertree (Strategic Decisions Group, Menlo Park, CA 94025).

Summary

Decision analysis presents a potentially effective method for objectively making pharmacoeconomic decisions based on probable outcomes and costs. Healthcare practitioners, both clinical and managerial, should find this a useful alternative in coping with decision-making situations brought on by diagnosis-related groups and other forms of cost-containment. It should assist in determining which alternative decision is the most cost-effective in a given situation. Thus, another useful aid has been added to the healthcare system repertoire of decision-making skills.

References

1. Ledley RS, Lusted LB. Reasoning foundations of medical diagnosis. *Science* 1959;*130*:9-21.
2. Lusted LB. Decision making in patient management. *N Engl J Med* 1971; *284*:416-24.

3. McNeil BJ, Keeler E, Adelstein SJ. Primer on certain elements of medical decision making. *N Engl J Med* 1975;*293*:221-51.

4. Kassirer JP. The principles of clinical decision making: an introduction to decision analysis. *Yale J Biol Med* 1976;*49*:149-64.

5. Kassirer JP, Moskowitz AJ, Lau J, Pauker SG. Decision analysis: a progress report. *Ann Intern Med* 1987;*106*:275-91.

6. Raiffa H. Decision analysis: introductory lectures under uncertainty. Reading, MA: Addison-Wesley Publishing, 1968.

7. Plante DA, Kassirer JP, Zarin DA, Pauker SG. Clinical decision consultation service. *Am J Med* 1986;*80*:1169-76.

8. Weinstein MC, Fineberg HV, eds. Clinical decision analysis. Philadelphia: WB Saunders, 1980.

9. Drummond MF, Stoddart GL, Torrance GW. Methods for the economic evaluation of health care programmes. Oxford: Oxford Medical Publications, 1987.

10. Barr JT, Schumacher GE. Applying decision analysis in therapeutic drug monitoring: using the receiver-operating characteristic curves in comparative evaluations. *Clin Pharm* 1986;*5*:239-46.

11. Tversky A, Kahneman D. Judgement under uncertainty; heuristics and biases. *Science* 1974;*185*:1124-31.

12. Weinstein MC, Fineberg FV. Clinical decision analysis. Philadelphia: WB Saunders, 1980:168-83.

13. Barza M, Pauker SG. The decision to biopsy, treat, or wait in suspected herpes encephalitis. *Ann Intern Med* 1980;*92*:641-9.

14. Clemens JD, Ransohoff DF. A quantitative assessment of pre-dental antibiotic prophylaxis for patients with mitral-valve prolapse. *J Chronic Dis* 1984; *37*:531-44.

15. Hedges JR, Lowe RA. Streptococcal pharyngitis in the emergency department: analysis of therapeutic strategies. *Am J Emerg Med* 1986;*4*:107-15.

16. Hillner BE, Centor RM. What a difference a day makes: a decision analysis of adult streptococcal pharyngitis. *J Gen Intern Med* 1987;*2*:242-8.

17. Oster G, Tuden RL, Colditz GA. A cost-effectiveness analysis of prophylaxis against deep-vein thrombosis in major orthopedic surgery. *JAMA* 1987; *257*:203-8.

18. Pauker SG. Coronary artery surgery: the use of decision analysis. *Ann Intern Med* 1976; *85*:8-18.

19. Rose DN, Schechter CB, Fahs MC, Silver AL. Tuberculosis prevention: cost-effectiveness analysis of isoniazid chemoprophylaxis. *Am J Prev Med* 1988;*4*:102-9.

20. Shapiro M, Schoenbaum SC, Tager IB, Munoz A, Polk BF. Benefit-cost analysis of antimicrobial prophylaxis in abdominal and vaginal hysterectomy. *JAMA* 1983;*249*:1290-4.

21. Stern RS, Pass TM, Komaroff AL. Topical versus systemic agent treatment for papulopustular acne: a cost-effectiveness analysis. *Arch Dermatol* 1984; *120*:1571-8.

22. Washington AE, Browner WS, Korenbrot CC. Cost-effectiveness of combined treatment for endocervical gonorrhea: considering co-infection with *Chlamydia trachomatis*. *JAMA* 1987;*257*:2056-60.

23. Weinstein MC, Read JL, MacKay DN, et al. Cost-effective choice of antimicrobial therapy for serious infections. *J Gen Intern Med* 1986;*1*:351-63.

24. Gottlieb JE, Pauker SG. Whether or not to administer amphotericin to an immunosuppressed patient with hematologic malignancy and undiagnosed fever. *Med Decis Making* 1981;*1*:75-93.

25. Plante DA, Pauker SG. Enterococcal endocarditis and penicillin allergy: which drug for the bug? *Med Decis Making* 1983;*3*:81-109.

26. Cuchural GJ, Levey AS, Pauker SG. Kidney failure or cancer: should immunosuppression be continued in a transplant patient with malignant melanoma? *Med Decis Making* 1984;*4*:83-107.

27. Eraker SA, Sasse L. The serum digoxin test and digoxin toxicity: a Bayesian approach to decision making. *Circulation* 1981;*64*:409-20.

28. Schumacher GE, Barr JT. Applying decision analysis in therapeutic drug monitoring: using decision trees to interpret serum theophylline concentrations. *Clin Pharm* 1986;*5*:325-33.

29. Reves RR, Johnson PC, Erisson CD, DuPont HL. A cost-effectiveness comparison of the use of antimicrobial agents for treatment or prophylaxis of travelers' diarrhea. *Arch Intern Med* 1988;*148*:2421-7.

30. Tsevat J, Durand-Zaleski I, Pauker SG. Cost-effectiveness of antibiotic prophylaxis for dental procedures in patients with artificial joints. *Am J Public Health* 1989;*79*:739-43.

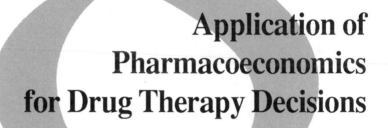

8

Application of
Pharmacoeconomics
for Drug Therapy Decisions

Jane T. Osterhaus
JoLaine R. Draugalis

he consequence of healthcare's spiraling costs is that a greater premium than ever before has been placed on employing all available healthcare resources as efficiently and effectively as possible. Efficiency and effectiveness must be demonstrated to Congress, taxpayers, third-party payers, and patients.[1] The demand for such information is evidenced by the proposed Medicare rules regarding criteria and procedures for making medical services coverage decisions that relate to healthcare technology:

> . . .We propose that HCFA and Medicare contractors consider the cost-effectiveness of a service when making coverage decisions. We believe considerations of cost are relevant in deciding whether to expand or continue coverage of technologies, particularly in the context of the current explosion of high-cost medical technologies. We believe that a disciplined effort to assess systematically the cost-effectiveness of technologies under coverage review will be useful. Cost-effectiveness means having improved health outcomes from Medicare patients that justify additional expenditures.[2]

A common interest among healthcare providers should be the patient. Yet, the interests tend to diverge rather than converge. This is demonstrated by our inability to measure and understand the effect of choices of patients, payers, and practitioners on the patients' functioning and well-being. Without such information, the bottom line as far as healthcare goods and services are concerned will continue to be costs.[3]

Along with other medical care goods and services, drugs are a form of healthcare technology that experienced significant inflation during the 1980s. As governments and other healthcare payers attempt to stretch their healthcare dollars, interest in evaluations that will contribute to the efficiency of the drug therapy decision process, (i.e., pharmacoeconomics), will rise. The demand for economic impact statements and outcome measures creates opportunities and presents challenges to practitioners to develop, collect, analyze, and interpret data and present pharmacoeconomic information. But where does pharmacoeconomics "fit in" with regular science? It should not be construed as an attempt to replace existing clinical trials, but rather looked on as an evaluative science, designed to improve the information base for clinical and policy decisions.[4]

Pharmacoeconomic research may be applied at many stages during the drug therapy decision process. In fact, it can be a very useful tool long before a drug is approved for use by the FDA. Pharmaceutical manufacturers recognize the need to avoid devoting enormous resources to development of a drug that does not provide a competitive advantage.[5] Competitive advantage in the current healthcare environment may be defined as a drug that is cost-effective. Cost-effective can mean a drug that is less costly and at least as effective as an alternative; more effective and more costly than an alternative, but improved health outcomes justify additional expenditures; or less effective and less costly than an existing alternative, but a viable alternative for some patients.[2]

The potential for an investigational new drug to leave the laboratory is a function of its expected safety and efficacy, which are both factors comprised of several specific measures or evaluations (e.g., toxicology, adverse reactions, teratogenicity, pharmacology). An additional factor worth considering is the expected pharmacoeconomics of the investigational drug. That factor also would be comprised of specific evaluations such as the societal and individual costs of the illness for which the drug is indicated, the costs and consequences of existing treatment methods, and the impact of the disease and existing treatments on patient quality-of-life (QOL). Having such information very early in the development of a drug would help reduce uncertainties and contribute to the knowledge base used to decide whether to further evaluate a treatment via prospective clinical trials. Cost-efficacy and QOL components can be incorporated into appropriate Phase III studies to provide additional information regarding a drug's impact on patient outcome. If such parameters are applied systematically to all new treatment candidates, the scientific basis of drug therapy decision-making will increase substantially.[4]

Cost-efficacy and QOL components from Phase III clinical trials may give an indication of the best outcomes to expect from treatment. After a drug is approved for use, pharmacoeconomic applications should continue in order to observe the actual economic and QOL impact of the treatment. As experience with the drug is gained in "real-world" settings, it is important to monitor actual patient outcomes and cost-effectiveness to determine the differences between that expected from clinical trials and that observed in actual practice. A macro or micro focus can be used in such cases, depending on whether one is concerned with a societal or nonsocial perspective. At the macro level, cost-benefit analysis attempts to maximize societal health, considering cost constraints. At the micro level, the traditional drug therapy decision process attempts to maximize the individual's health, regardless of cost. Cost-benefit analysis might be at odds with the clinical decision analysis but, historically, has not interfered with the treatment decisions made. Cost-benefit analyses conducted at the national or public policy level have been sufficiently removed from the individual practitioner/patient interaction; there has been neither conflict nor amalgamation between the two approaches.[6]

However, this situation is being changed by various healthcare reforms that give healthcare providers responsibility for treatment decisions tied into a framework of societally based incentives and competition (such as diagnosis-related groups and relative value units). National rates now are used to determine the appropriate length of stay for hospitalized patients. Decisions at the individual patient level are still based on clinically defined good practice; however, cost considerations and national norms also receive a significant amount of attention.

The clinical research management model suggested by Bruxton demonstrates the importance of pharmacoeconomic research to the practitioner in the cost-conscious healthcare environment.[1,6] The model combines the criteria of the traditional clinical management model, but is based on economically justifiable clinical protocols and aimed at maximizing benefit to a specifically defined group of patients. All of the costs falling within a clinically focused budget are considered, and the patients' values and preferences are taken into account. The expected outcome would determine the extent of care provided. For example, after a drug has been approved by the FDA, a pharmacoeconomic analysis may indicate that the drug is cost-effective for certain patient groups. Such a research finding is valuable from a pharmaceutical company's perspective because it identifies the target market. It also helps practitioners make efficient decisions on therapy because they can combine that information with the information they already have regarding the patient's status. The clinical research management model provides clinicians with opportunities for economic and QOL evaluation, and allows a provider to consider the possible trade-offs between alternative treatments.[1,6]

Healthcare has been described as a bundle of goods and services.[7] Human resources typically are combined with medical technology to diagnose or treat a disease. One component without the others may be useless, or even dangerous, so it is important to ensure that the components are bundled appropriately. When evaluating various healthcare activities, it is important to consider all of the components (goods and services) used to provide a certain service or procedure from the various perspectives of interest. When pharmacoeconomic tools are used to evaluate a particular treatment, the evaluations should include an assessment of the drug-related services provided by practitioners. Such services are one of the necessary components of the treatment process.

Drug use evaluation is considered by many to be an important service provided by pharmacists.[8-10] Ideally, that value should be translated into patient and financial outcomes. It is easy to demonstrate that by using fewer drugs, one can reduce a drug budget, but that begs the question: What about the total system budget? How does a drug use evaluation program affect a state Medicaid budget? What happens to the patients? Furthermore, as drug use evaluation expands, it is likely that, in addition to concentrating on inappropriately prescribed therapy and overprescribing, use of the most cost-effective therapy will also be important. A high degree of sophistication will be required in order to make such a determination fairly, considering patient factors, disease factors, and other issues.

Drug formulary services and pharmacy and therapeutics committees also have been viewed as a positive means of reducing drug budgets and have had some value in encouraging drug therapy cost considerations,[11,12] but they do not provide incentives to take into account overall medical costs, nor do they necessarily consider all consequences, such as potential drug interactions, adverse reactions, and treatment response rates. Conducting cost-effectiveness studies allows an evaluation of total costs and consequences from various perspectives. Croog et al. found that three antihypertensive medications that achieved similar blood pressure control differed notably in their effects on functioning and well-being.[13] Information regarding such treatment effects will be important to consider when therapeutic substitution issues are discussed.

Relationship to Clinical Pharmacy Services

The value of pharmacy services, like many other healthcare services, may be questioned because people do not understand the services' benefits. Garnett noted: "The biggest mistake of the clinical [pharmacy] movement in hospitals was the failure to initially generate cost-effectiveness data. Too often physicians' acceptance of clinical pharmacists' services was adequate"[as a means of justifying continuing the service].[14]

The American College of Clinical Pharmacy has disseminated a position statement that presented an overview of the documentation available to support the economic value of clinical pharmacy services. In addition, methodologic shortcomings of past evaluations were pointed out, as well as points to consider when undertaking economic evaluations of clinical pharmacy services. Finally, a plan was proposed regarding the need for more documentation of the economic value of clinical services. An appendix listed studies that have been conducted.[15]

MacKeigan and Bootman discussed the purpose and methodology of cost-benefit analysis (CBA) and cost-effectiveness analysis (CEA) in evaluating clinical pharmacy services. They reviewed applications of the techniques used in 22 evaluative studies published between 1978 and mid-1987. Their major conclusions were that "CBA and CEA had not been extensively adopted in the evaluation of clinical pharmacy services and that the studies which have been done are lacking in rigor." Only full economic evaluations were considered in the review. That is, studies must have examined output benefits (or effectiveness) in addition to reporting input costs. The majority of the studies were cost-minimization analyses.[16]

There may be a fine line between some service applications and specific drug-therapy decisions resulting from pharmacoeconomic inquiry. For instance, cost-justification of a pharmacokinetic dosing service and the economic assessment of aminoglycoside therapy could be interrelated.

Bootman and McGhan described economic analytic techniques applied to the evaluation of therapeutic drug monitoring services. It was stated that future funding for these types of programs will go to those administrators able to justify their services by increasing drug-use control, improving the cost-effectiveness of drug therapy, and increasing productivity. Methods for determining costs and benefits were discussed.[17] In a study designed to assess the cost-benefit of an aminoglycoside monitoring service, the benefits were appropriateness and economic efficiency of aminoglycoside therapy. The relationship between clinical decision-making and evaluation of the service was indicated by the reduction in cost per course of therapy being primarily due to preferential use of gentamicin over tobramycin. This recommendation was due to clinical considerations as well as acquisition costs.[18]

As clinical pharmacy and pharmacoeconomics expand to the community and outpatient sectors, it is vital to remember that the major decision makers in healthcare have changed; the perspectives of administrators, payers, and patients are now as important as those of physicians. Pharmacoeconomic studies, therefore, must evaluate more than one perspective. If pharmacy wants to establish or expand services, in community and/or inpatient settings, the appropriateness of those services will have to be documented. The services must be considered valuable from a variety of perspectives. A positive impact on patient outcome, justified by the resources expended to provide the care, has to be demonstrated.

Limitations

It is important to be aware of the limitations as well as the usefulness of pharmacoeconomic analyses. The questions of cost must always be followed by the inquiry "to whom?" A study conducted from different perspectives may generate different results. Remember to ask, "Cost-effective from whose perspective?"[19]

Pharmacoeconomic evaluations provide the tools to analyze the economic results of alternative drug therapy decisions. They do not, however, provide unequivocal selection. There is always an element of uncertainty regarding the etiology of disease, and diagnostic and curative techniques. Additionally, a consensus may never be reached on such issues as the value of the discount rate, reducing uncertainty, estimating in the face of uncertainty, and taking into account the concept of equity. Sensitivity analysis examines such uncertain events under different assumptions, indicating the confidence one can place in their results, thereby reducing but not totally eliminating uncertainty. This is why such analyses require systematic and rigorous approaches. Those involved in drug-therapy decision making must understand the strengths and weaknesses of approaches to this emerging field and use the tools in the appropriate manner.[19,20]

Given all the evidence of the increasing importance of pharmacoeconomic analyses, it is important that the pharmacy practitioner be able to critically read the published works in the area. Decisions must be made regarding methodologies employed, validity of conclusions, and ability to generalize findings.

Assessing the Pharmacoeconomic Literature

Reading and using the results from pharmacoeconomic studies is much like using the results of any research in that a critical assessment of methods, assumptions, limitations, etc., is required. Moreover, criteria specific to economic evaluations such as discounting, sensitivity analysis, and incremental analysis are also important. The following criteria were assembled based on guidelines and checklists that have been published.[21-24]

This inquiry list is not provided to make readers hypercritical and unaccepting of articles. Very few, if any, reports would meet these criteria in total. However, as a guide they can be useful in determining whether it is worth the reader's time to continue, and if so, whether results and conclusions are deemed valid based on the methodologies employed. Some journals stipulate section headings, length, content requirements, etc. This may need to be considered when critiquing a report. Many of these are important when assessing any type of research report/article. Another caveat is the misuse of terminology in the pharmacoeconomic literature. For example, cost-benefit has been inappropriately used as a synonym for a cost-analysis or cost-minimization study. Additionally, cost-saving is not always equal to cost-effective, yet many authors have equated the two.[25] Chapter 3 contains critical information on economic variables to integrate with this checklist. Finally, not all categories will apply to each and every report.

Criteria for Evaluating Pharmacoeconomic Studies

1. TITLE

    a. Is it interesting?
    b. Is it informative?

2. ABSTRACT OR SUMMARY

    a. Are the following addressed: purpose, methodology, results, conclusions?
    b. If appropriate, are hypotheses clearly stated?
    c. If the results were valid, would they be useful in your institution/practice site?

3. INTRODUCTION

    a. Are the problem statement and resultant study questions clearly and precisely stated?

    b. Where appropriate, are the hypotheses to be tested stated in a testable form?

    c. Whose perspective is considered? Society, healthcare payer, patient, healthcare provider?

4. LITERATURE REVIEW

    a. Is the relationship of the study question clearly related to previous research?

    b. Is the significance of the inquiry discussed with resultant justification of the research?

5. METHODOLOGY

    a. Alternatives
- What alternatives are compared? Were the options described in sufficient detail?
- What is the primary concern? Most beneficial use of limited resources (CBA)? Least costly way to achieve an objective (CEA)? Demonstrating equivalency in comparative groups (cost-minimization analysis)? Natural units adjusted for quality-of-life (cost-utility analysis)?
- Are the appropriate alternatives compared? Does the analysis compare the new entity against a current standard? Are all relevant alternatives considered?

    b. Economic variables
- Are all relevant costs and consequences considered? If an important variable is excluded, is justification given?
- Which variables are included? Medical resources (basic and intermediate), nonmedical resources, productive capacity, effectiveness variables (clinical indicators, cases treated, life-years saved, other), health status variables (quality-adjusted life-year)?
- How are the costs and consequences measured or counted?
- How are the costs and consequences valued? Acquisition costs, hospital services (per diem, room and board plus ancillary, charges, cost-to-charge ratio), wages (plus benefits)?
- What is the source of data? Medical records, data collection form (retrospective, concurrent)?
- Are the options compared in terms of additional costs and additional benefits? (incremental analysis)

    c. Subjects

- Are the sampling frame and method described?
- If applicable, are sources of sampling bias considered?

d. Instruments
- Is the instrument valid for the study setting and research questions?
- Does the instrument yield reliable observations for the study setting and research questions?
- If a nonstandardized instrument is being utilized, what information is given regarding its development?

e. Design
- Is the design appropriate when considering the literature review and research hypotheses?
- Is the design internally valid?
- Is the description complete enough to allow replication?

f. Assumptions and limitations
- Are assumptions and limitations clearly stated?

g. Analysis
- How are data analyzed?
- If utilized, are statistical methods appropriate?

6. RESULTS

a. Are the results of the analysis clearly presented?
b. Is there sufficient evidence to answer the study questions?
c. If utilized, are the reported statistics relevant to the research hypotheses?
d. Is the pictorial representation of data complete and readily understood?

7. SENSITIVITY ANALYSIS

a. Is a sensitivity analysis conducted for variables that may not be measured with certainty?
b. Do the results change when factors are varied?

8. DISCOUNTING

a. Are future costs and consequences discounted?
b. Is any rationale given for the rate chosen?

9. DISCUSSION AND CONCLUSIONS

a. Are results in light of the original problem statement(s)?
b. Are results compared to previous inquiries?
c. Are conclusions substantiated?
d. Are generalizations appropriate?
e. Are implications and recommendations presented?

10. OVERALL CONSIDERATIONS

a. Is the report organized and clearly written?

b. Is there an unbiased, impartial attitude portrayed?

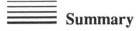 **Summary**

As we are confronted with the reality that there is a limit to resources, we must become increasingly concerned that services provided are efficient and effective.[1,20] Some health systems are only now recording why interventions are done and/or how well they worked. The tools used in pharmacoeconomic research that measure health outcomes for the patient as a "bottom line" need to be incorporated in ambulatory and hospital practices.

The major health-related advances of earlier research in conquering polio and tuberculosis had clear benefits; more younger people lived. The benefits of current research tend to help older people live longer. The gains are less pronounced because it will cost more to keep a retired person alive and there had been some debate about whether a year's life in old age is worth as much as a year for a younger person.[1] At the same time, enhancing daily functioning and well-being is an increasingly advocated goal in patient treatment of chronic conditions.[26] The need for QOL assessments are highlighted by such considerations.

The pharmacoeconomist has an opportunity to educate healthcare professionals and others, such as corporate benefits administrators. If economic and QOL research are to be conducted and interpreted appropriately, the concept of considering the total costs of treating an illness, not just concentrating on each component separately, must be explained. The term quality-of-life, and the implications of changes in QOL must be understood. Patient outcome measures should serve to reunite the divergent views of many practitioners who have the patient's best interest at heart.

Drug evaluation has been characterized as the best established and understood paradigm to evaluate healthcare technologies.[4] Yet, there is more uncertainty than consensus regarding the clinical use of drugs. Pharmacoeconomic analysis "fits in" the drug therapy decision process as an evaluative clinical science that can help reduce uncertainty about probabilities and patient value of drug therapy outcomes. This will improve the information base for clinical decisions. These types of inquiry provide excellent collaborative opportunities, particularly between the clinical pharmacy and pharmacy administration disciplines.

Pharmacoeconomic analysis should not be seen as a mechanism for deciding automatically on the allocation of funds, but as a structure for helping to weigh advantages and disadvantages. Since the adoption of a new technology may be limited by a lack of cost-effectiveness and QOL information, it is most advantageous to initiate such studies as early as possible in the drug development process.

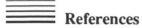 References

1. Pharmaceuticals and economics, future considerations. *Scrip* 1989;*1462*:5-9. (A report of a conference on "Measuring the Benefits of Medicines, the future agenda," sponsored by the Office of Health Economics in London.)

2. Medicare program's criteria and procedures for making medical services coverage decisions that relate to health care technology. *Fed Reg* 1989;*54*:4302-18.

3. Ellwood PM. A technology of patient experience. *N Engl J Med* 1988;*313*:1549-56.

4. Wennberg JE. Improving the medical decision-making process. *Health Aff* 1988; 7(Spring):99-106.

5. Wilson CF, Hall WF. Challenges of drug discovery, global development and marketing in the 1990s. *Drug News Perspect* 1989;2:380-1.

6. Health economics and the pharma industry. *Scrip* 1989;*1381*:12-3.

7. Schlegel JF. Rebundling health care. *Am Pharm* 1988;*NS28*:378-83.

8. Hepler CD, Strand LM. Opportunities and responsibilities in pharmaceutical care. *Am J Hosp Pharm* 1990;*47*:533-43.

9. Lomaestro BM, Lesar TS. DUE of ticarcillin and clavulanate potassium: determining appropriate and cost-effective therapeutic options. *Hosp Formul* 1988;*23*:909-13.

10. Chrischilles EA, Helling DK, Aschoff CR. Effect of clinical pharmacy services on the quality of family practice physician prescribing and medication costs. *DICP Ann Pharmacother* 1989;23:417-21.

11. Segal R, Pathak DS. Formulary decision making: identifying factors that influence P&T committee drug evaluations. *Hosp Formul* 1988;*23*:174-8.

12. Andrews JD, Hafting S. Financial impact of formulary revision on second generation cephalosporins. *Can J Hosp Pharm* 1988;*41*:125-7.

13. Croog SH, Levine S, Testa MA, et al. The effects of antihypertensive therapy on the quality of life. *N Engl J Med* 1986;*314*:1657-64.

14. Garnett WR. The final frontier: clinical pharmacy practice in community pharmacy settings. *Am J Pharm Educ* 1989;*53*:313-4.

15. Willett MS, Bertch KE, Rich DS, Ereshefsky L. Prospectives on the economic value of clinical pharmacy services: a position statement of the American College of Clinical Pharmacy. *Pharmacotherapy* 1989;9:45-56.

16. MacKeigan LD, Bootman JL. A review of cost-benefit and cost-effectiveness analyses of clinical pharmacy services. *J Pharm Market Manage* 1988;2:63-84.

17. Bootman JL, McGhan WF. Cost-benefit of therapeutic drug monitoring. In: Taylor WJ, Diers Caviness MH, eds. A textbook for the clinical application of therapeutic drug monitoring. Irving, TX: Abbott Laboratories Diagnostic Division, 1986:67-84.

18. Kimelblatt BJ, Bradbury K, Chodoff L, Aggour T, Mehl B. Cost-benefit analysis of an aminoglycoside monitoring service. *Am J Hosp Pharm* 1986;*43*:1205-9.

19. Office of Technology Assessment. The implications of cost effectiveness analysis of medical technology. Background paper #1: methodological issues and literature review. Washington, DC: United States Congress, 1980.

20. Wasylenki D. The importance of economic evaluations (editorial). *Can J Psychiatry* 1989;*34*:631.

21. Ward MJ, Fetler ME. Research Q & A: what guidelines should be followed in critically evaluating research reports? *Nurs Res* 1979;*28*:120-6.

22. Sackett DL. How to read clinical journals: Part I. Why to read them and how to start reading them critically. *Can Med Assoc J* 1981;*124*:555-8.

23. Drummond M, Smith GT, Wells N. Economic evaluation in the development of medicines. London: Office of Health Economics, 1988:28-9.

24. Larson LN. Pharmacoeconomics and formulary decisions. *Dyn Health Care* 1989;*1*:11-4.

25. Draugalis JR, Bootman JL, Larson LN, McGhan WF. Current concepts—pharmacoeconomics. Kalamazoo, MI: The Upjohn Company, 1989:7.

26. Stewart AL, Greenfield S, Hays RD, et al. Functional status and well-being of patients with chronic conditions. *JAMA* 1989;*262*:907-13.

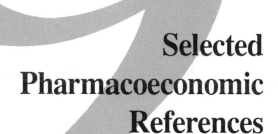

Selected
Pharmacoeconomic
References

J. Lyle Bootman

he following is a compilation of selected references for various medical disease states. There was no attempt by the authors to develop a comprehensive list. The purpose was to identify for our readers selected research articles currently in print. Hopefully, these articles will assist interested people in pursuing further the application of pharmacoeconomic methodologies to the review of existing literature as well as the development of new primary literature.

Arthritis, Osteoporosis, Psoriasis

Brooks RG, Brown MG, Marsh JM, Woodbury JF. Costs of managing patients at a Canadian rheumatic disease unit. *J Rheumatol* 1981;*8*:937-48.

Stern RS, Thibodeau LA, Kleinerman RA, Parrish JA, Fitzpatrick TB, Bleich HL. Effect of methoxsalen photochemotherapy on cost of treatment for psoriasis: an example of technological assessment. *JAMA* 1981;*245*:1913-8.

Pullar T, Capell HA, Millar A, Brooks RG. Alternative medicine: cost and subjective benefit in rheumatoid arthritis. *Br Med J [Clin Res]* 1982;*285*:1629-31.

Ehrlich GE. Social, economic, psychologic, and sexual outcomes in rheumatoid arthritis. *Am J Med* 1983;*75(6A)*:27-34.

Stone CE. The lifetime economic costs of rheumatoid arthritis. *J Rheumatol* 1984;*11*:819-27.

Stern RS. Long-term use of psoralens and ultraviolet A for psoriasis: evidence for efficacy and cost savings. *J Am Acad Dermatol* 1986;*14*:520-6.

Avioli LV. Socio-economic costs of osteoporosis and changing patterns. *Ann Chir Gynaecol* 1988;77:168-72.

Champion GD. A perspective on the cost-effectiveness and risks of nonsteroidal anti-inflammatory drug therapy. *Med J Aust* 1988;*149*:346-9.

Ross PD, Wasnich RD, Maclean CJ, Hagino R, Vogel JM. A model for estimating the potential costs and savings of osteoporosis prevention strategies. *Bone* 1988;*9*:337-47.

Stern RS. The benefits, costs and risks of topical tar preparations in the treatment of psoriasis: considerations of cost-effectiveness. *Ann Acad Med Singapore* 1988;*17*:473-6.

Thompson MS, Read JL, Hutchings HC, Paterson M, Harris ED Jr. The cost effectiveness of auranofin: results of a randomized clinical trial. *J Rheumatol* 1988;*15*:35-42.

Hawkey C. Nonsteroidal anti-inflammatory drugs in patients with peptic ulcer disease: rarely justified in terms of cost or patient benefit. *Br Med J* 1989;*298*:177-8.

Helewa A, Bombardier C, Goldsmith CH, Menchions B, Smythe HA. Cost-effectiveness of inpatient and intensive outpatient treatment of rheumatoid arthritis: a randomized, controlled trial. *Arthritis Rheum* 1989;*32*:1505-14.

Levy E. Cost analysis of osteoporosis related to untreated menopause. *Clin Rheumatol* 1989; *8*(suppl 2):76-82.

Cancer

Hartunian NS, Smart CN, Thompson MS. The incidence and economic costs of cancer, motor vehicle injuries, coronary heart disease and stroke: a comparative analysis. *Am J Public Health* 1980;*70*:1249-60.

Baird SB. Economic realities in the treatment and care of the cancer patient. *Top Clin Nurs* 1981;*2*(4):67-80.

Rice DP, Hodgson TA. Social and economic implications of cancer in the United States. *Vital Health Stat* 1981;*3*(20):1-43.

Hodgson TA. Economic cost of cancer in the United States, 1980. *Prog Clin Biol Res* 1983; *132E*:373-82.

Carroll PR, Williams RD, Kim MJ, Dombrovskis S. Mitomycin C reused: an in vitro cost-effectiveness study. *J Urol* 1984;*132*:583-6.

Wetchler SJ. Treatment of cervical intraepithelial neoplasia with the CO_2 laser: laser versus cryotherapy: a review of effectiveness and cost. *Obstet Gynecol Surv* 1984;*39*:469-73.

Rees GJG. Cost-effectiveness in oncology (letter). *Lancet* 1985;*2*:28.

Lea MS, Stahlgren LH. Is resection appropriate for adenocarcinoma of the pancreas? A cost-benefit analysis. *Am J Surg* 1987;*154*:651-4.

Macdonald EA. Cost-effectiveness of cancer chemotherapy: risks/benefit ratio: socio-economic and ethical considerations. *Cancer Treat Rev* 1987;*14*:345-50.

Parashos PJ, Dugan WM Jr, Fry MW. Continuous infusion metoclopramide: clinical trials. *Prog Clin Biol Res* 1987;*248*:303-11.

Goodwin PJ, Feld R, Evans WK, Pater J. Cost-effectiveness of cancer chemotherapy: an economic evaluation of a randomized trial in small-cell lung cancer. *J Clin Oncol* 1988;*6*: 1537-47.

Greenberg ER, Chute CG, Stukel T, et al. Social and economic factors in the choice of lung cancer treatment: a population-based study in two rural states. *N Engl J Med* 1988; *318*:612-7.

Markman M. An argument in support of cost-effectiveness analysis in oncology. *J Clin Oncol* 1988;*6*:937-9.

Stoll BA. Balancing cost and benefit in treatment of late cancer. *Lancet* 1988;*1*:579-80.

Timothy AR, Brewin T, Chamberlain J, et al. Cost versus benefit in nonsurgical management of patients with cancer. *Br Med J [Clin Res]* 1988;*297*:471-2.

Gilewski T, Vogelzang NJ. Cost-effectiveness and reimbursement issues in renal cell carcinoma. *Semin Oncol* 1989;*16*(suppl 1):20-6.

Macdonald JS. Continuous low-dose infusion of fluorouracil: is the benefit worth the cost? *J Clin Oncol* 1989;*7*: 412-4.

Ozer H, Golomb HM, Zimmerman H, Spiegel RJ. Cost-benefit analysis of interferon alfa-2b in treatment of hairy cell leukemia. *J Natl Cancer Inst* 1989;*81*:594-602.

Robinson ME, Leonard JR. A chemotherapy self learning package: a cost-effective method. *J Nurs Staff Dev* 1989;*5*(3):144.

Shibley L, Brown M, Schuttinga J, Rothenberg M, Whalen J. Cisplatin-based combination chemotherapy in the treatment of advanced-stage testicular cancer: cost-benefit analysis. *J Natl Cancer Inst* 1990;*82*:186-92.

Dental

Manau C, Cuenca E, Martinez-Carretero J, Sallaras L. Economic evaluation of community programs for the prevention of dental caries in Catalonia, Spain. *Community Dent Oral Epidemiol* 1987;*15*:297-300.

Kraal JH. Cost-effectiveness analysis of periodontal disease control (letter). *J Dent Res* 1988; *67*:611.

O'Rourke CA, Attrill M, Holloway PJ. Cost appraisal of a fluoride tablet program to Manchester primary schoolchildren. *Community Dent Oral Epidemiol* 1988;*16*:341-4.

Tsevat J, Durand-Zaleski I, Pauker SG. Cost effectiveness of antibiotic prophylaxis for dental procedures in patients with artificial joints. *Am J Public Health* 1989;*79*:739-43.

Diabetes

Fagin JA, Litwak L, Gutman RA. Economic realities of home blood glucose monitoring (letter). *Lancet* 1983;*2*:682-3.

Jonsson B. Diabetes—the cost of illness and the cost of control: an estimate for Sweden, 1978. *Acta Med Scand* 1983;*671*(suppl):19-27.

Krosnick A. Economic impact of type II diabetes mellitus. *Prim Care* 1988;*15*:423-32.

Javitt JC, Canner JK, Sommer A. Cost effectiveness of current approaches to the control of retinopathy in type I diabetics. *Ophthalmology* 1989;*96*:255-64.

≡ Gastrointestinal Disease

Oberle MW, Merson MH, Islam MS, Rahman AS, Huber DH, Curlin G. Diarrheal disease in Bangladesh: epidemiology, mortality averted, and costs at a rural treatment center. *Int J Epidemiol* 1980;*9*:341-8.

Culver AJ, Maynard AK. Cost-effectiveness of duodenal ulcer treatment. *Soc Sci Med* 1981; *15C*:3-11.

Geweke J, Weisbrod BA. Clinical evaluation versus economic evaluation: the case of a new drug. *Med Care* 1982;*20*:821-30.

Jensen DM. Health and economic aspects of peptic ulcer disease. *Am J Med* 1984;77(5B):8-14.

Lerman SJ, Shepard DS, Cash RA. Treatment of diarrhea in Indonesian children: what it costs and who pays for it. *Lancet* 1985;*2*:651-4.

Nyren O, Adami HO, Gustavsson S, Loof L, Nyberg A. Social and economic effects of nonulcer dyspepsia. *Scand J Gastroenterol* 1985;*109*(suppl):41-7.

Jensen DM. Economic and health aspects of peptic ulcer disease and H_2-receptor antagonists. *Am J Med* 1986;*81*(4B):42-8.

Bolin TD. Effectiveness and cost of antiulcer medications (letter). *Med J Aust* 1987;*147*:418- 20.

Guerrant RL, Wanke CA, Barrett LJ, Schwartzman JD. A cost effective and effective approach to the diagnosis and management of acute infectious diarrhea. *Bull NY Acad Med* 1987;*63*:484-99.

McLean AJ, Harcourt DM, McCarthy PG, Dudley FJ, McNeil JJ. Relative effectiveness and costs of antiulcer medications as a basis for rational prescribing. *Med J Aust* 1987; *146*:431-3, 436-8, 442.

Robinson IG. Effectiveness and cost of antiulcer medications (letter). *Med J Aust* 1987; *147*:206-7.

Tuggle DW, Hoelzer DJ, Tunell WP, Smith EI. The safety and cost-effectiveness of polyethylene glycol electrolyte solution bowel preparation in infants and children. *J Pediatr Surg* 1987;*22*:513-5.

Howden CW. Maintenance treatment with H_2-receptor antagonists in patients with peptic ulcer disease: rarely justified in terms of cost or patient benefit. *Br Med J* 1988;*297*:1393-4.

Jensen DM. Economic assessment of peptic ulcer disease treatments. *Scand J Gastroenterol* 1988;*146*(suppl):214-24.

Reves RR, Johnson PC, Ericsson CD, DuPont HL. A cost-effectiveness comparison of the use of antimicrobial agents for treatment or prophylaxis of travelers' diarrhea. *Arch Intern Med* 1988;*148*:2421-7.

Singh KP, Jain AK, Singh RH, Gupta JP. Relative potency and cost-effectiveness of different antacids: in vitro study. *J Assoc Physicians India* 1988;*36*:323-5.

Hawkey C. Nonsteroidal anti-inflammatory drugs in patients with peptic ulcer disease: rarely justified in terms of cost or patient benefit. *Br Med J* 1989;*298*:177-8.

Macdonald JS. Continuous low-dose infusion of fluorouracil: is the benefit worth the cost? *J Clin Oncol* 1989;*7*:412-4.

Nolly RJ, Skoutakis VA. Cost considerations of intravenously administered histamine$_2$-receptor antagonists. *DICP Ann Pharmacother* 1989;*23*(suppl):S23-8.

Sonnenberg A. Costs of medical and surgical treatment of duodenal ulcer. *Gastroenterology* 1989;*96*:1445-52.

Heart Disease

Hartunian NS, Smart CN, Thompson MS. The incidence and economic costs of cancer, motor vehicle injuries, coronary heart disease, and stroke: a comparative analysis. *Am J Public Health* 1980;*70*:1249-60.

Hauser RG. The cost of tachyarrhythmia management. *Arch Mal Coeur* 1985;*78*:35-7.

Laffel GL, Fineberg HV, Braunwald E. A cost-effectiveness model for coronary thrombolysis/ reperfusion therapy. *J Am Coll Cardiol* 1987;*10*(5 suppl B):79B-90B.

Olsson G, Levin LA, Rehnqvist N. Economic consequences of postinfarction prophylaxis with beta blockers: cost-effectiveness of metoprolol. *Br Med J [Clin Res]* 1987;*294*:339-42.

Oster G, Epstein AM. Cost-effectiveness of antihyperlipemic therapy in the prevention of coronary heart disease. *JAMA* 1987;*258*:2381-7.

Evans RW, Manninen DL. Economic impact of cyclosporine in transplantation. *Transplant Proc* 1988;*20*(suppl 3):49-62.

Goldman L, Sia ST, Cook EF, Rutherford JD, Weinstein MC. Costs and effectiveness of routine therapy with long-term beta-adrenergic antagonists after acute myocardial infarction. *N Engl J Med* 1988;*319*:152-7.

Hall JP, Heller RF, Dobson AJ, Lloyd DM, Sanson-Fisher RW, Leeder SR. A cost-effectiveness analysis of alternative strategies for the prevention of heart disease. *Med J Aust* 1988;*148*: 273-7.

Kinosian BP, Eisenberg JM. Cutting into cholesterol. Cost-effective alternatives for treating hypercholesterolemia. *JAMA* 1988;*259*:2249-54.

Klevay LM. Cost-effectiveness of antihyperlipemic therapy (letter). *JAMA* 1988;*259*:1811.

McIntosh HD. How to integrate cost-effective measures into your practice. Perspectives, epilogue and caveat. *J Am Coll Cardiol* 1988;*12*:1119-21.

Olsson G. Economic aspects of beta-blocker therapy following myocardial infarction (letter). *J R Soc Med* 1988;*81*:242.

Seminar on Preventive Cardiology. How to integrate cost-effective measures into your practice. *J Am Coll Cardiol* 1988;*12*:1089-145.

Steinberg EP, Topol EJ, Sakin JW, et al. Cost and procedure implications of thrombolytic therapy for acute myocardial infarction. *J Am Coll Cardiol* 1988;*12*(6 suppl A):58A-68A.

Underhill SL. Economic issues: a challenge to cardiovascular nurses. *Prog Cardiovasc Nurs* 1988;*3*:37-8.

Vermeer F, Simoons ML, deZwaan C, et al. Cost-benefit analysis of early thrombolytic treatment with intracoronary streptokinase: 12-month follow up report of the randomized multicentre trial conducted by the Interuniversity Cardiology Institute of The Netherlands. *Br Heart J* 1988;*59*:527-34.

Berger GM. Cost-effective treatment of hyperlipidaemia (letter). *S Afr Med J* 1989;*76*:387.

Chapekis AT, Burek K, Topol EJ. The cost:benefit ratio of acute intervention for myocardial infarction: results of a prospective, matched pair analysis. *Am Heart J* 1989;*118*(5 pt 1):878-82.

Lezaun R, Brugada P, Smeets J, et al. Cost-benefit analysis of medical versus surgical treatment of symptomatic patients with accessory atrioventricular pathways. *Eur Heart J* 1989; *10*:1105-9.

Martens LL, Rutten FF, Erkelens DW, Ascoop CA. Cost effectiveness of cholesterol-lowering therapy in The Netherlands: simvastatin versus cholestyramine. *Am J Med* 1989; *87*(4A):54S-8S.

Mizgal HF. Contemporary treatment of acute myocardial infarction and unstable angina: cost effectiveness (editorial). *Can J Cardiol* 1989;*5*:127-8.

White DH, Clinton PK. Cost-effective treatment of hyperlipidemia (letter). *S Afr Med J* 1989; *75*:596.

Hypertension

McCarron DA, Hare LE, Walker BR. Therapeutic and economic controversies in antihypertensive therapy. *J Cardiovasc Pharmacol* 1984;*6*(suppl 5):S837-40.

Steinwachs DM. Cost-effectiveness analysis: role in evaluation of alternatives for improving high blood pressure control. *Md State Med J* 1984;*33*:225-7.

Stason WB. Opportunities for improving the cost-effectiveness of antihypertensive treatment. *Am J Med* 1986;*81*(6C):45-9.

Oster G, Huse DM, Delea TE, Savage DD, Colditz GA. Cost effectiveness of labetalol and propranolol in the treatment of hypertension among blacks. *J Natl Med Assoc* 1987;*79*: 1049-55.

Stason WB. Economics in hypertension management: cost and quality trade-offs. *J Hypertens* 1987;*5*(suppl):S55-9.

Malcolm LA, Kawachi I, Jackson R, Bonita R. Is the pharmacological treatment of mild to moderate hypertension cost effective in stroke prevention? *N Z Med J* 1988;*101*:167-71.

Miller JA, Hansen PC. Economic costs and benefits of treating mild hypertension: results from a cross-sectional model. *N Z Med J* 1988;*101*:623-5.

Seedat YK. Do newer agents confer added cost-benefit in the management of hypertension? (editorial) *S Afr Med J* 1988;*74*:543-4.

Blaufox MD. Cost-effectiveness of nuclear medicine procedures in renovascular hypertension. *Semin Nucl Med* 1989;*19*:116-21.

Burns R. Cost-effectiveness in the treatment of hypertension. *Clin Geriatr Med* 1989;*5*:829-40.

Edgar MA, Schnieden H. The economics of mild hypertension programs. *Soc Sci Med* 1989;*28*:211-22.

Grimm RH Jr. Epidemiological and cost implications of antihypertensive treatment for the prevention of cardiovascular disease. *J Hum Hypertens* 1989;*3*(suppl 2):55-60.

Harlan WR. Economic considerations that influence health policy and research. *Hypertension* 1989;*13*(5 pt 2):1158-63.

Russell LB. Cost-effectiveness of antihypertensive treatment. General considerations. *Hypertension* 1989;*13*(5 pt 2):1141-4.

Edelson JT, Weinstein MD, Tosteson AN, Williams L, Lee TH, Goldman L. Long-term cost-effectiveness of various initial monotherapies for mild to moderate hypertension. *JAMA* 1990;*263*:407-13.

Infectious Disease

PROPHYLAXIS OF INFECTIOUS DISEASE

Antimicrobials

Lidwell OM. The cost implications of clean air systems and antibiotic prophylaxis in operations for total joint replacement. *Infect Control* 1984;*5*:36-7.

Ford LC. Cost of antibiotic prophylaxis in cesarean section. *Drug Intell Clin Pharm* 1986; *20*:592-3.

Gladen HE. Cost-effective aminoglycoside therapy in surgical patients. *Am J Med* 1986; *80*(6B): 228-33.

Briggs GG, Moore BR, Bahado-Singh R, Lange S, Bogh P, Garite TJ. Cost-effectiveness of cefonicid sodium versus cefoxitin sodium for the prevention of postoperative infections after nonelective cesarean section. *Clin Pharm* 1987;*6*:718-21.

Duff P. Prophylactic antibiotics for cesarean delivery: a simple cost-effective strategy for prevention of postoperative morbidity. *Am J Obstet Gynecol* 1987;*157*(4 pt 1):794-8.

Ford LC, Hammil HA, Lebherz TB. Cost-effective use of antibiotic prophylaxis for cesarean section. *Am J Obstet Gynecol* 1987;*157*:506-10.

Glazier HS. Cost-effectiveness of cefonicid versus cefoxitin prophylaxis for cesarean section (letter). *Clin Pharm* 1987;*6*:923-4.

Hay JW, Daum RS. Cost-benefit analysis of two strategies for prevention of *Haemophilus influenzae* type B infection. *Pediatrics* 1987;*80*:319-29.

Jorup-Ronstrom C, Britton S. Recurrent erysipelas: predisposing factors and costs of prophylaxis. *Infection* 1987;*15*:105-6.

Patriarca PA, Arden NH, Koplan JP, Goodman RA. Prevention and control of type A influenza infections in nursing homes. Benefits and costs of four approaches using vaccination and amantadine. *Ann Intern Med* 1987;*107*:732-40.

Ciola B. A readily adaptable, cost-effective method of infection control for dental radiography. *J Am Dent Assoc* 1988;*117*:349.

D'Angelo GL, Ogilvie-Harris DJ. Septic arthritis following arthroscopy, with cost/benefit analysis of antibiotic prophylaxis. *Arthroscopy* 1988;*4*:10-4.

Daschner FD. How cost-effective is the present use of antiseptics? *J Hosp Infect* 1988;*11*(suppl A):227-35.

Davey PG, Duncan ID, Edward D, Scott AC. Cost-benefit analysis of cephradine and mezlocillin prophylaxis for abdominal and vaginal hysterectomy. *Br J Obstet Gynaecol* 1988;*95*:1170-7.

Persson U, Montgomery F, Carlsson A, Lindgren B, Ahnfelt L. How far does prophylaxis against infection in total joint replacement offset its cost? *Br Med J [Clin Res]* 1988;*296*: 99-102.

Platt R, Lehr JL, Marino S, Munoz A, Nash B, Raemer DB. Safe and cost-effective cleaning of pressure-monitoring transducers. *Infect Control Hosp Epidemiol* 1988;*9*:409-16.

Buhaug H, Skjeldestad FE, Backe B, Dalen A. Cost effectiveness of testing for chlamydial infections in asymptomatic women. *Med Care* 1989;*27*:833-41.

Chin A, Gill MA, Ito MK, et al. Cost-analysis of two clindamycin dosing regimens. *DICP Ann Pharmacother* 1989;*23*:980-3.

Daschner F. Cost-effectiveness in hospital infection control—lessons for the 1990s. *J Hosp Infect* 1989;*13*:325-36.

Lawrence VA, Gafni A, Gross M. The unproven utility of the preoperative urinalysis: economic evaluation. *J Clin Epidemiol* 1989;*42*:1185-92.

MacCormack CP, Snow RW, Greeenwood BM. Use of insecticide-impregnated bed nets in Gambian primary health care: economic aspects. *Bull WHO* 1989;*67*:209-14.

Miller PJ, Farr BM, Gwaltney JM Jr. Economic benefits of an effective infection control program: case study and proposal. *Rev Infect Dis* 1989;*11*:284-8.

Platt R, Polk BF, Murdock B, Rosner B. Prevention of catheter-associated urinary tract infection: a cost-benefit analysis. *Infect Control Hosp Epidemiol* 1989;*10*:60-4.

Immunizations

Golden M, Shapiro GL. Cost benefit analysis of alternative programs of vaccination against rubella in Israel. *Public Health* 1984;*98*:179-90.

Hinman AR, Koplan JP. Pertussis and pertussis vaccine. Reanalysis of benefits, risks and costs. *JAMA* 1984;*251*:3109- 13.

Koplan JP. Benefits, risks and costs of immunization programs. *Ciba Found Symp* 1985;*110*: 55-68.

Corrao G, Zotti C, Tinivella F, Moirashi Ruggenini A. HBV prevaccination screening in hospital personnel: cost-effectiveness analysis. *Eur J Epidemiol* 1987;*3*:25-9.

Creese AL, Dominguez-Uga MA. Cost-effectiveness of immunization programs in Colombia. *Bull Pan Am Health Organ* 1987;*21*:377-94.

Davis RM, Markowitz LE, Preblud SR, Orenstein WA, Hinman AR. A cost-effectiveness analysis of measles outbreak control strategies. *Am J Epidemiol* 1987;*126*:450-9.

Hankins DG, Ebert KD, Siebold CM, Fuller TK, Frascone RJ, Campion BC. Hepatitis B vaccine and hepatitis B markers: cost-effectiveness of screening prehospital personnel. *Am J Emerg Med* 1987;*5*:205-6.

Hay JW, Daum RS. Cost-benefit analysis of two strategies for prevention of *Haemophilus influenzae* type b infection. *Pediatrics* 1987;*80*:319-29.

Jonsson B. Cost-benefit analysis of hepatitis B vaccination. *Postgrad Med J* 1987;*63*(suppl 2):27-32.

Lahaye D, Strauss P, Baleux C, van Ganse W. Cost-benefit analysis of hepatitis B vaccination. *Lancet* 1987;*2*:441-3.

Morrison AJ Jr, Hunt EH, Atuk NO, Schwartzman JD, Wenzel RP. Rabies pre-exposure prophylaxis using intradermal human diploid cell vaccine: immunologic efficacy and cost-effectiveness in a university medical center and a review of selected literature. *Am J Med Sci* 1987;*293*:293-7.

Patriarca PA, Arden NH, Koplan JP, Goodman RA. Prevention and control of type A influenza infections in nursing homes. Benefits and costs of four approaches using vaccination and amantadine. *Ann Intern Med* 1987;*107*:732-40.

Arevalo JA, Washington AE. Cost-effectiveness of prenatal screening and immunization for hepatitis B virus. *JAMA* 1988;*259*:365-9. Erratum appears in *JAMA* 1988;*260*:478.

Dominguez-Uga MA. Economic analysis of the vaccination strategies adopted in Brazil in 1982. *Bull Pan Am Health Organ* 1988;*22*:250-68.

Evans DB, Hensley MJ, O'Connor SJ. Influenza vaccination in Australia: a review of the economic evidence for policy recommendations. *Med J Aust* 1988;*149*:540-3.

Hutchison BG, Stoddart GL. Cost-effectiveness of primary tetanus vaccination among elderly Canadians. *Can Med Assoc J* 1988;*139*:1143-51.

Little RF, Brenner ER, Macera CA, Jackson KL. Cost-effective prevaccine screening of hepatitis B infection in hospital workers: a seroepidemiological study. *J S C Med Assoc* 1988;*84*:409-13.

McConnochie KM, Hall CB, Barker WH. Lower respiratory tract illness in the first two years of life: epidemiologic patterns and costs in a suburban pediatric practice. *Am J Public Health* 1988;*78*:34-9.

Stephenne J. Recombinant versus plasma-derived hepatitis B vaccines: issues of safety, immunogenicity and cost-effectiveness. *Vaccine* 1988;*6*:299-303.

Tong MJ, Co RL, Marci RD, Michaelson PM, Ortega G. A cost comparison analysis for screening and vaccination of hospital personnel with high- and low-prevalence hepatitis B virus antibodies in California. *Infect Control Hosp Epidemiol* 1988;*9*(2):66-71.

Weber DJ, Rutala WA, Parham C. Impact and costs of varicella prevention in a university hospital. *Am J Public Health* 1988;*78*:19-23.

Carducci A, Avio CM, Bendinelli M. Cost-benefit analysis of tetanus prophylaxis by a mathematical model. *Epidemiol Infect* 1989;*102*:473-83.

Fisher SA, Hennink M. Screening before immunization against hepatitis B—is it cost-effective? (letter) *S Afr Med J* 1989;*76*:387.

Hicks RA, Cullen JW, Jackson MA, Burry VF. Hepatitis B virus vaccine. Cost-benefit analysis of its use in a children's hospital. *Clin Pediatr* 1989;*28*:359-65.

McKee CM, Dinsmore WW. Hepatitis B immunization in Northern Ireland: an epidemiological and economic analysis. *Ir Med J* 1989;*82*(2):83-7.

Muckle TJ. Cost-effectiveness of primary tetanus vaccination among elderly Canadians (letter). *Can Med Assoc J* 1989;*140*:586-7.

Phonboon K, Shepard DS, Ramaboot S, Kunasol P, Preuksaraj S. The Thai expanded program on immunization: role of immunization sessions and their cost-effectiveness. *Bull WHO* 1989;*67*:181-8.

Tsevat J, Durand-Zaleski I, Pauker SG. Cost effectiveness of antibiotic prophylaxis for dental procedures in patients with artificial joints. *Am J Public Health* 1989;*79*:739-43.

TREATMENT

Foster GE, Bourke JB, Bolwell J, et al. Clinical and economic consequences of wound sepsis after appendectomy and their modification by metronidazole or povidone iodine. *Lancet* 1981;*1*:769-71.

Smith DL, Brauer WA. Comparative costs of diagnosis and treatment in acute pharyngitis. *South Med J* 1981;*74*:332-4.

McGowan JE Jr. Cost and benefit: a critical issue for hospital infection control. *Am J Infect Control* 1982;10:100-8.

Rapp RP, Bannon CL, Bivins BA. The influence of dose frequency and agent toxicity on the cost of parenteral antibiotic therapy. *Drug Intell Clin Pharm* 1982;*16*:935-8.

Bell RE, Yoder BA, Ackerman NB Jr, Null DM Jr, DeLemos RA. Military neonatal transport and intensive care: effective and cost-effective. *Milit Med* 1984;*149*:143-5.

Stern RS, Pass TM, Komaroff AL. Topical versus systemic agent treatment for papulopustular acne: a cost-effective analysis. *Arch Dermatol* 1984;*120*:1571-8.

Bosso JA, Huckendubler Stephenson SE, Herbst JJ. Feasibility and cost savings of intravenous administration of aminoglycosides in outpatients with cystic fibrosis. *Drug Intell Clin Pharm* 1985;*19*:52-4.

Dawson CR, Schachter J. Strategies for treatment and control of blinding tachoma: cost-effectiveness of topical or systemic antibiotics. *Rev Infect Dis* 1985;*7*:768-73.

Dixon RE. Economic costs of respiratory tract infections in the United States. *Am J Med* 1985; *78*(6B): 45-51.

Faro S. Patient cost in the treatment of postsurgical female pelvic infection. *Am J Med* 1985; *78*(6B):165-9.

Lerman SJ, Shepard DS, Cash RA. Treatment of diarrhea in Indonesian children: what it costs and who pays for it. *Lancet* 1985;*2*:651-4.

Shandera WX, Taylor JP, Betz TG, Blake PA. An analysis of economic costs associated with an outbreak of typhoid fever. *Am J Public Health* 1985;*75*:71-3.

Hill WL. Economic evaluation of pharmacologic therapy. *Drug Intell Clin Pharm* 1986; *20*:594-6.

Washington AE, Arno PS, Books MA. The economic cost of pelvic inflammatory disease. *JAMA* 1986;*255*:1735-8.

Bailey RR. Cost-benefit considerations in the management of uncomplicated urinary tract infections in sexually active women. *N Z Med J* 1987;*100*:680-3.

Carlson KJ. Cost-effectiveness analysis of single-dose therapy of urinary tract infection compared to conventional treatment. *Eur Urol* 1987;*13*(suppl 1):45-7.

Fox GN. Cost-effectiveness and the management of pharyngitis (letter). *JAMA* 1987;*257*:2167-9.

Guerrant RL, Wanke CA, Barrett LJ, Schwartzman JD. A cost effective and effective approach to the diagnosis and management of acute infectious diarrhea. *Bull N Y Acad Med* 1987; *63*:484-99.

Holmberg SD, Solomon SL, Blake PA. Health and economic impacts of antimicrobial resistance. *Rev Infect Dis* 1987;*9*:1065-78.

Jorup-Ronstrom C, Britton S. Recurrent erysipelas: predisposing factors and costs of prophylaxis. *Infection* 1987;*15*:105-6.

Mathews A, Bailie GR. Clinical pharmacokinetics, toxicity and cost effectiveness analysis of aminoglycosides and aminoglycoside dosing services. *J Clin Pharm Ther* 1987; *12*:273-91.

Phaosavasdi S, Snidvongs W, Thasanapradit P, et al. Cost-benefit analysis of diagnosis and treatment of syphilis in pregnant women. *J Med Assoc Thai* 1987;70:90-5.

Quintiliani R, Cooper BW, Briceland LL, Nightingale CH. Economic impact of streamlining antibiotic administration. *Am J Med* 1987;82(4A):391-4.

Ramirez-Ronda C, Colon M, Saavedra S, Sabbaj J, Corrado ML. Treatment of urinary tract infection with norfloxacin: analysis of cost. *Am J Med* 1987;82(6B):75-8.

Washington AE, Browner WS, Korenbrot CC. Cost-effectiveness of combined treatment for endocervical gonorrhea. *JAMA* 1987;257:2056-60.

Washington AE, Johnson RE, Sanders LL Jr. *Chlamydia trachomatis* infections in the United States: what are they costing us? *JAMA* 1987;257:2070-2.

Wise GJ, Goldman WM, Goldberg PE, Rothenberg RG. Miconazole: a cost-effective antifungal genitourinary irrigant. *J Urol* 1987;138:1413-5.

Bailie GR, Mathews A. Cost-benefit analysis of aminoglycoside use without a kinetic dosing service (letter). *Drug Intell Clin Pharm* 1988;22:80-1.

Caldwell JR, Seligson RW. Economic stresses of AIDS: lessons for the United States and Florida. *J Fla Med Assoc* 1988;75:449-52.

Callahan CW Jr. Cost-effectiveness of antibiotic therapy for otitis media in a military pediatric clinic. *Pediatr Infect Dis J* 1988;7:622-5.

Chamberlain TM, Lehman ME, Groh MJ, Munroe WP, Reinders TP. Cost analysis of a home intravenous antibiotic program. *Am J Hosp Pharm* 1988;45:2341-5.

Kane RE, Jennison K, Wood C, Black PG, Herbst JJ. Cost savings and economic considerations using home intravenous antibiotic therapy for cystic fibrosis patients. *Pediatr Pulmonol* 1988;4:84-9.

Katz BP, Danos CS, Quinn TS, Caine V, Jones RB. Efficiency and cost-effectiveness of field follow-up for patients with *Chlamydia trachomatis* infection in a sexually transmitted diseases clinic. *Sex Transm Dis* 1988;15:11-6.

Leigh DA. Economic implications of oral treatment replacing parenteral therapy in antimicrobial chemotherapy. *Chemioterapia* 1988;7:400-5.

Penin GB, Ehrenkranz NJ. Priorities for surveillance and cost-effective control of postoperative infection. *Arch Surg* 1988;123:1305-8.

Reves RR, Johnson PC, Ericsson CD, DuPont HL. A cost-effectiveness comparison of the use of antimicrobial agents for treatment or prophylaxis of travelers' diarrhea. *Arch Intern Med* 1988;148:2421-7.

Sanders WE Jr. Efficacy, safety, and potential economic benefits of oral ciprofloxacin in the treatment of infections. *Rev Infect Dis* 1988;10:528-43.

Scitovsky AA. The economic impact of AIDS in the United States. *Health Aff* 1988;7(4):32-45.

Sochalski A, Sullman S, Andriole VT. Cost-effectiveness study of cefotetan versus cefoxitin and cefotetan versus combination antibiotic regimens. *Am J Surg* 1988;155(5A):96-101.

Weiss JC, Melman ST. Cost-effectiveness in the choice of antibiotics for the initial treatment of otitis media in children: a decision analysis approach. *Pediatr Infect Dis J* 1988;7:23-6.

Guglielmo BJ, Brooks GF. Antimicrobial therapy: cost-benefit considerations. *Drugs* 1989; 38:473-80.

Joesoef MR, Remington PL, Jiptoherijanto PT. Epidemiological model and cost-effectiveness analysis of tuberculosis treatment programs in Indonesia. *Int J Epidemiol* 1989;*18*:174-9.

Lawrence VA, Gafni A, Gross M. The unproven utility of the preoperative urinalysis: economic evaluation. *J Clin Epidemiol* 1989;*42*:1185-92.

Lopez AM, Keirns S, Wang H, Goldberg RN. A reliable and cost-effective neonatal aminoglycoside administration system. *Neonatal Netw* 1989;*7*(4):7-10.

McKenna JP, Chamovitz BN. Cost-effective treatment of pseudomembranous colitis. *Am Fam Physician* 1989;*39*(4):74,78.

Grayson ML, McNeil JJ, Lucas CR. Economic and educational status of zidovudine recipients in Melbourne (letter). *Med J Aust* 1990;*152*:49-50.

O'Leary MP. Economic considerations in management of complicated urinary tract infections. *Urology* 1990;*35*(suppl 1):22-4

Mental Illness

Muller CF, Caton CL. Economic costs of schizophrenia: a postdischarge study. *Med Care* 1983;*21*:92-104.

Andrews G, Hall W, Goldstein G, Lapsley H, Bartels R, Silove D. The economic costs of schizophrenia. Implications for public policy. *Arch Gen Psychiatry* 1985;*42*:537-43.

Hall W, Goldstein G, Andrews G, Lapsley H, Bartels R, Silove D. Estimating the economic costs of schizophrenia. *Schizophr Bull* 1985;*11*:598-610.

Edlund MJ, Swann AC. The economic and social costs of panic disorder. *Hosp Commun Psychiatry* 1987;*38*:1277-9, 1288.

Harwood HJ, Hubbard RL, Collins JJ, Rachal JV. The costs of crime and the benefits of drug abuse treatment: a cost-benefit analysis using TOPS data. *NIDA Res Monogr* 1988;*86*:209-35.

Woodfield A. Economic cost of alcohol-related health care in New Zealand: an interpretive comment. *Br J Addict* 1988;*83*:1031-5.

Wray N, Brody B, Bayer T, et al. Withholding medical treatment from the severely demented patient: decisional processes and cost implications. *Arch Intern Med* 1988;*148*:1980-4.

Ferencckik B, Mathew RJ. Alcoholism treatment. Cost and effectiveness favor ambulatory programs. *N C Med J* 1989;*50*:195-8.

Hayashida M, Alterman AI, McLellan AT, et al. Comparative effectiveness and costs of inpatient and outpatient detoxification of patients with mild-to-moderate alcohol withdrawal syndrome. *N Engl J Med* 1989;*320*:358-65.

Lobeck F, Traxler WT, Bobinet DD. The cost-effectiveness of a clinical pharmacy service in an outpatient mental health clinic. *Hosp Community Psychiatry* 1989;*40*:643-5.

Wasylenki DA. The importance of economic evaluations (editorial, comment). *Can J Psychiatry* 1989;*34*:631-2.

Nutrition

Hinsdale JG, Lipkowitz GS, Pollock TW, Hoover EL, Jaffe BM. Prolonged enteral nutrition in malnourished patients with nonelemental feeding: reappraisal of surgical technique, safety, and costs. *Am J Surg* 1985;*149*:334-8.

Twomey PL, Patching SC. Cost-effectiveness of nutritional support. *JPEN J Parenter Enteral Nutr* 1985;*9*:3-10.

Eisenberg JM, Glick H, Hillman AL, et al. Measuring the economic impact of perioperative total parenteral nutrition: principles and design. *Am J Clin Nutr* 1988;*47*(suppl):382-91.

Horn E. Iron and folate supplements during pregnancy: supplementing everyone treats those at risk and is cost-effective. *Br Med J* 1988;*297*:1325,1327.

Reilly JJ Jr, Hull SF, Albert N, Waller A, Bringardener S. Economic impact of malnutrition: a model system for hospitalized patients. *JPEN J Parenter Enteral Nutr* 1988;*12*:371-6.

Pulmonary Disease

Johnson DE, Munson DP, Thompson TR. Effect of antenatal administration of betamethasone on hospital costs and survival of premature infants. *Pediatrics* 1981;*68*:633-7.

Oster G, Huse DM, Delea TE, Colditz GA. Cost-effectiveness of nicotine gum as an adjunct to physician's advice against cigarette smoking. *JAMA* 1986;*256*:1315-8.

Alpers JH. Domiciliary oxygen: the cost-benefit dilemma (editorial). *Med J Aust* 1987;*146*:62-3.

Clausen JL. Self-administration of bronchodilators. Cost effective? (editorial) *Chest* 1987; *91*:475.

Jasper AC, Mohsenifar Z, Kahan S, Goldberg HS, Koerner SK. Cost-benefit comparison of aerosol bronchodilator delivery methods in hospitalized patients. *Chest* 1987;*91*:614-8.

Mounla NA, Baassiri GM. Cost effectiveness of neonatal inhalation therapy. *Middle East J Anesthesiol* 1987;*9*:77-81.

Howard P. Cost effectiveness of oxygen therapy. *Eur Respir J* 1989;*2*(suppl):637s-9s.

Joesoef MR, Remington PL, Jiptoherijanto PT. Epidemiological model and cost-effectiveness analysis of tuberculosis treatment programs in Indonesia. *Int J Epidemiol* 1989;*18*:174-9.

M'elot C, Lejeune P, Leeman M, Moraine JJ, Naeije R. Prostaglandin E_1 in the adult respiratory distress syndrome. Benefit for pulmonary hypertension and cost for pulmonary gas exchange. *Am Rev Respir Dis* 1989;*139*:106-10.

Thromboembolism

Rooke TW, Osmundson PJ. Heparin and the in-hospital management of deep venous thrombosis: cost considerations. *Mayo Clin Proc* 1986;*61*:198-204.

Graor RA, Young JR, Risius B, Ruschhaupt WF. Comparison of cost effectiveness of streptokinase and urokinase in the treatment of deep vein thrombosis. *Ann Vasc Surg* 1987; *1*:524-8.

Laffel GL, Fineberg HV, Braunwald E. A cost-effectiveness model for coronary thrombolysis/reperfusion therapy. *J Am Coll Cardiol* 1987;*10*(5 suppl B):79B-90B.

Oster G, Tuden RL, Colditz GA. A cost-effectiveness analysis of prophylaxis against deep-vein thrombosis in major orthopedic surgery. *JAMA* 1987;*257*:203-8.

Oster G, Tuden RL, Colditz GA. Prevention of venous thromboembolism after general surgery. Cost-effectiveness analysis of alternative approaches to prophylaxis. *Am J Med* 1987; *82*:889-99.

Paiement GD, Bell D, Wessinger SJ, Harris WH. The Otto Aufranc Award paper. New advances in the prevention, diagnosis, and cost effectiveness of venous thromboembolic disease in patients with total hip replacement. *Hip* 1987;*94*:94-119.

Schwarzman P, Rottman SJ. Prehospital use of heparin locks: a cost-effective method for intravenous access. *Am J Emerg Med* 1987;*5*:475-7.

Dacey LJ, Dow RW, McDaniel MD, Walsh DB, Zwolak RM, Cronenwett JL. Cost-effectiveness of intraarterial thrombolytic therapy. *Arch Surg* 1988;*123*:1218-23.

Richton-Hewett S, Foster E, Apstein CS. Medical and economic consequences of a blinded oral anticoagulant brand change at a municipal hospital. *Arch Intern Med* 1988;*148*:806-8.

Steinberg EP, Topol EJ, Sakin JW, et al. Cost and procedure implications of thrombolytic therapy for acute myocardial infarction. *J Am Coll Cardiol* 1988;*12*(6 suppl A):58A-68A.

Vermeer F, Simoons ML, deZwaan C, et al. Cost-benefit analysis of early thrombolytic treatment with intracoronary streptokinase: 12-month follow-up report of the randomized multicenter trial conducted by the Interuniversity Cardiology Institute of the Netherlands. *Br Heart J* 1988;*59*:527-34.

Williams JT, Palfrey SM. Cost effectiveness and efficacy of below knee against above knee graduated compression stockings in the prevention of deep vein thrombosis. *Phlebologie* 1988;*41*:809-11.

Ansell JE, Hamke AK, Holden A, Knapic N. Cost-effectiveness of monitoring warfarin therapy using standard versus capillary prothrombin times. *Am J Clin Pathol* 1989;*91*:587-9.

Cole MG. Flushing heparin locks: is saline flushing really cost-effective? *J Intraven Nurs* 1989; *12*(1 suppl):S23-9.

Meister FL, McLauglin TF, Tenney RD, Sholkoff SD. Urokinase. A cost-effective alternative treatment of superior vena cava thrombosis and obstruction. *Arch Intern Med* 1989; *149*:1209-10.

Miscellaneous

Norton WL. Chemonucleolysis versus surgical discectomy. Comparison of costs and results in workers' compensation claimants. *Spine* 1986;*11*:440-3.

DeAngelis C. How effective is cost-effective analysis? (editorial). *J Pediatr* 1988;*112*:574-5.

Evans RW, Manninen DL. Economic impact of cyclosporine in transplantation. *Transplant Proc* 1988;*20*(3 suppl 3):49-62.

Hollenberg JP, Subak LL, Ferry JJ Jr, Bussel JB. Cost-effectiveness of splenectomy versus intravenous gamma globulin in treatment of chronic immune thrombocytopenic purpura in childhood. *J Pediatr* 1988;*112*:530-9.

Kane RE, Jennison K, Wood C, Black PG, Herbst JJ. Cost savings and economic consider-ations using home intravenous antibiotic therapy for cystic fibrosis patients. *Pediatr Pulmonol* 1988;*4*:84-9.

Silfvenius H. Economic costs of epilepsy—treatment benefits. *Acta Neurol Scand Suppl* 1988; *117*:136-54.

Simmons JW, Avant WS Jr, Demski J, Parisher D. Determining successful pain clinic treatment through validation of cost effectiveness. *Spine* 1988;*13*:342-4.

Tabibian N. Cost-effective methods of treating ascites. *Am Fam Physician* 1988;*37*:141-6.

Weiner CP, Renk K, Klugman M. The therapeutic efficacy and cost-effectiveness of aggressive tocolysis for premature labor associated with premature rupture of the membranes. *Am J Obstet Gynecol* 1988;*159*:216-22.

Blenkinsopp A. Cost-benefit of self-prescribing (letter). *Lancet* 1989;*1*:1393.

Emery DD, Schneiderman LJ. Cost-effectiveness analysis in health care. *Hastings Cent Rep* 1989;*19*(4):8-13.

Fischer AJ, Yellowlees PM. Prevention of the Wernicke-Korsakoff syndrome in Australia: a cost-benefit analysis. *Med J Aust* 1989;*150*:311-3, 317.

Gelvin JB, Boen TM. Dosage cost-analysis in glaucoma management. *J Am Optom Assoc* 1989;*60*:768-70.

Goodburn E, Mattosinho S, Monge P, Waterston T. Cost-benefit of self prescribing (letter). *Lancet* 1989;*2*:281.

Hillman BJ, Kahan JP, Neu SP, Hammons GT. Clinical trials to evaluate cost-effectiveness. *Invest Radiol* 1989;*24*:167-71 .

Huse DM, Oster G, Killen AR, Lacey MJ, Colditz GA. The economic costs of non-insulin-dependent diabetes mellitus. *JAMA* 1989;*262*:2708-13.

Jones L, Neiswender JA, Perkins M. PCA: patient satisfaction, nursing satisfaction and cost-effectiveness. *Nurs Manage* 1989;*20*:16-7.

Lipscomb J. Time preference for health in cost-effectiveness analysis. *Med Care* 1989;*27*(3 suppl):S233-53.

Moore FM, Simpson D. Cost-effective assays for use in monitoring carbamazepine, pheno-barbital, and phenytoin in serum. *Clin Chem* 1989;*35*:1782-4.

Pierce GF, Lusher JM, Brownstein AP, Goldsmith JC, Kessler CM. The use of purified clotting factor concentrates in hemophilia. Influence of viral safety, cost, and supply on therapy. *JAMA* 1989;*261*:3434-8.

Steele MA, Bess DT, Franse VL, Graber SE. Cost effectiveness of two interventions for re-ducing outpatient prescribing costs. *DICP Ann Pharmacother* 1989;*23*:497-500.

Index